Demos Surgical Pathology Guides

Prostate Pathology

DEBRA L. ZYNGER, MD
Director, Genitourinary Surgical Pathology
Associate Professor
Department of Pathology
The Ohio State University Medical Center
Columbus, Ohio

ANIL V. PARWANI, MD, PHD
Director, Pathology Informatics
Professor
Department of Pathology
University of Pittsburgh Medical Center
Pittsburgh, Pennsylvania

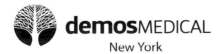

demosMEDICAL
New York

Visit our website at www.demosmedical.com

ISBN: 9781936287901
e-book ISBN: 9781617051524

Acquisitions Editor: Rich Winters
Compositor: diacriTech

Medicine is an ever-changing science. Research and clinical experience are continually expanding our knowledge, in particular our understanding of proper treatment and drug therapy. The authors, editors, and publisher have made every effort to ensure that all information in this book is in accordance with the state of knowledge at the time of production of the book. Nevertheless, the authors, editors, and publisher are not responsible for errors or omissions or for any consequences from application of the information in this book and make no warranty, expressed or implied, with respect to the contents of the publication. Every reader should examine carefully the package inserts accompanying each drug and should carefully check whether the dosage schedules mentioned therein or the contraindications stated by the manufacturer differ from the statements made in this book. Such examination is particularly important with drugs that are either rarely used or have been newly released on the market.

Library of Congress Cataloging-in-Publication Data

Zynger, Debra L., author.
  Prostate pathology / Debra L. Zynger, Anil V. Parwani.
      p. ; cm. — (Demos surgical pathology guides)
  Includes bibliographical references and index.
  ISBN 978-1-936287-90-1 — ISBN 978-1-61705-152-4 (e-book)
  I. Parwani, Anil V., author. II. Title. III. Series: Demos surgical pathology guides.
  [DNLM: 1. Prostatic Diseases—pathology. WJ 752]
  RC899
  616.6'507—dc23   2014010811

Special discounts on bulk quantities of Demos Medical Publishing books are available to corporations, professional associations, pharmaceutical companies, health care organizations, and other qualifying groups. For details, please contact:

Special Sales Department
Demos Medical Publishing, LLC
11 West 42nd Street, 15th Floor
New York, NY 10036
Phone: 800-532-8663 or 212-683-0072
Fax: 212-941-7842
E-mail: specialsales@demosmedical.com

Printed in the United States of America by Bang Printing.
14 15 16 17 / 5 4 3 2 1

Contents

Series Foreword

The field of surgical pathology has gained increasing relevance and importance over the years as pathologists have become more and more integrated into the health care team. To the need for precise histopathologic diagnoses has now been added the burden of providing our clinical colleagues with information that will allow them to assess the prognosis of the disease and predict the response to therapy. Pathologists now serve as key consultants in the patient management team and are responsible for providing critical information that will guide their therapy. With the progress gained due to the insights obtained from the application of newer diagnostic techniques, surgical pathology has become progressively more complex. As a result, diagnoses need to be more detailed and specific and the number of data elements required in the generation of a surgical pathology report have increased exponentially, making management of the information required for diagnosis cumbersome and sometimes difficult.

The past 15 years have witnessed an explosion of information in the field of pathology with a massive proliferation of specialized textbooks appearing in print. For the most part, such texts provide in-depth and detailed coverage of the various areas in surgical pathology. The purpose of this series is to bridge the gap between the major subspecialty texts and the large, double-volume general surgical pathology textbooks, by providing compact, single-volume monographs that will succinctly address the most salient and important points required for the diagnosis of the most common conditions. The series is organized following an organ-system format, with single volumes dedicated to individual organs. The volumes are divided on the basis of disease groups, including benign reactive, inflammatory, infectious or systemic conditions, benign neoplastic conditions, and malignant neoplasms. Each chapter consists of a bulleted list of the most pertinent clinical data related to the condition, followed by the most important histopathologic criteria for diagnosis, pertinent use of immunohistochemical stains and other ancillary techniques, and relevant molecular tests when available. This is followed by a section on differential diagnosis. References appear at the back of the volume. Each entity is illustrated with key, high-quality histological images that highlight the most salient and distinctive features that need to be recognized for the correct diagnosis.

These books are intended for the busy practicing pathologist, and for pathology residents and fellows in training who require an easy and simple overview of major diagnostic criteria and key points during the course of routine daily practice. The authors have been carefully chosen for their experience in the field and clarity of exposition in the various topics. It is hoped that this series will fulfill its purpose of providing quick and easy access to critical information for the busy practitioner or trainee, and that it will assist pathologists in their routine practice of the specialty.

Saul Suster, MD
Professor and Chairman
Department of Pathology
Medical College of Wisconsin
Milwaukee, Wisconsin

Preface

Prostate pathology is a field with a myriad of specialized nomenclature and evolving diagnoses as our understanding of the disease processes increases. Tissue examined by pathologists demands more rigorous attention to detail due to the PSA screening era producing diminishing tumor. Because pathologists are expected to make diagnoses on smaller and smaller tumors, knowledge of benign mimickers of cancer, ability to recognize the cancer features to detect rare glands of tumor, and understanding of immunohistochemical stains to corroborate a diagnosis of carcinoma are essential for the practicing pathologist.

This book has been designed to assist pathologists in diagnosing prostate specimens for their daily practice. An overview of prostate pathology is provided, highlighting the most important concepts throughout the text. A description of the normal prostate, with a review of structures that are essential to recognize is provided. The book is composed of three sections: Nonneoplastic conditions, premalignant conditions and prostate carcinoma, and mesenchymal, hematopoietic and secondary tumors. Nonneoplastic conditions address inflammation, atrophy, adenosis, hyperplasia, metaplasia, and other normal structures which can be confused with prostatic adenocarcinoma. Premalignant conditions and prostate carcinoma details high-grade prostatic intraepithelial neoplasia, prostatic adenocarcinoma including diagnostic features of carcinoma and Gleason grading, as well as other unusual types of carcinoma. Mesenchymal, hematopoietic and secondary tumors contains a succinct review of rarely encountered entities.

Each topic features headings including definition, clinical features, microscopic features, ancillary studies, and differential diagnosis. Text is provided in a concise, bulleted format for efficient and facile use by the reader with a focus on practical information. Text is followed by key images to point out the main diagnostic features of each entity. References are collated at the end of the volume.

We hope that this text will serve as an up to-date and convenient reference manual for practicing pathologists as well as pathologists in training.

Introduction: The Normal Prostate

DEFINITION
■ The normal prostate is composed of glands with an acinar and a basal cell layer surrounded by fibromuscular stroma.

MICROSCOPIC FEATURES
■ The outer layer of basal cells is characterized by flattened to low cuboidal cells with nuclei oriented parallel to the basement membrane (Figure 1). Nuclei are more blue to light purple in comparison to the inner acinar cells. In many glands, the basal cells may be difficult to visualize without the use of ancillary immunohistochemistry.

(text continued on page xii)

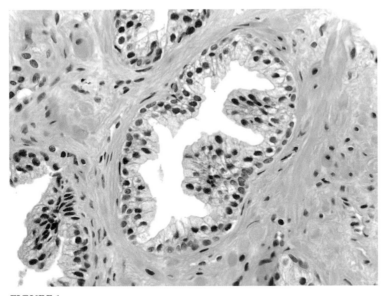

FIGURE 1

FIGURE 1   A normal prostate gland is composed of outer basal cells and an inner acinar layer.

- The inner secretory layer consists of a single to pseudostratified columnar layer with nuclei oriented perpendicular to the basement membrane. Nuclei are a darker purple compared to the outer basal cells. The cytoplasm is moderate to abundant, fluffy, and pale pink.
- Corpora amylacea, dense eosinophilic laminated secretions, are sometimes present within the lumen (Figure 2).

ANCILLARY STUDIES
- The basal cell markers, p63 (nuclear staining) and high molecular weight keratin (HMWK including CK5 or CK5/6) (cytoplasmic staining) highlight the basal cell layer present in nonneoplastic glands, high-grade prostatic intraepithelial neoplasia, and surrounding intraductal carcinoma. Basal cell markers are negative in prostate cancer and some nonneoplastic entities such as partial atrophy (Figures 3 and 4).
- Alpha-methylacyl-CoA racemase (AMACR or P504s) (granular cytoplasm staining) is expressed within prostatic adenocarcinoma and is variable within high-grade prostatic intraepithelial neoplasia and nonneoplastic lesions such as atrophy and adenosis (Figures 3 and 4).

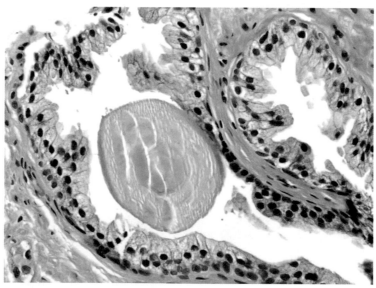

FIGURE 2

FIGURE 2 Within the lumen of a normal prostate gland, a corpora amylacea is seen.

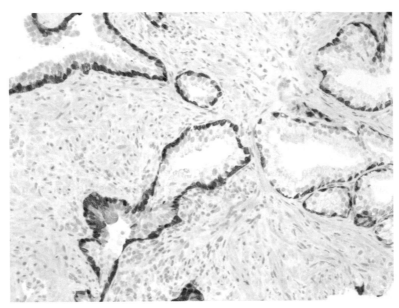

FIGURE 3

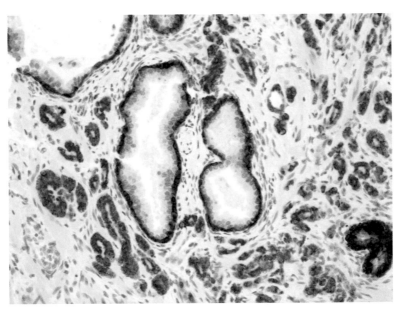

FIGURE 4

FIGURE 3 In normal glands, p63 (nuclear brown) and HMWK (cytoplasmic brown) are strongly positive while AMACR (cytoplasmic pink) is almost entirely absent.

FIGURE 4 Larger normal glands express p63 and HMWK (brown) and are negative for AMACR (pink) while smaller glands of prostatic adenocarcinoma invading between and around the nonneoplastic glands are positive for AMACR and are negative for p63 and HMWK.

Prostate Pathology

Nonneoplastic Conditions

1

INFLAMMATION

Acute Inflammation

DEFINITION
■ Acute inflammatory infiltrate involving the prostate.

CLINICAL FEATURES
■ Approximately half of prostate needle core biopsies contain acute inflammation which may be caused by blocked prostatic ducts/acini.
■ Acute inflammation is associated with serum prostate-specific antigen (PSA) elevation and for this reason may be relevant to document if identified.
■ The term "acute prostatitis" should be avoided as prostatitis implies clinical sequelae.

MICROSCOPIC FEATURES
■ Intraluminal and epithelial neutrophils are seen. Periglandular and stomal neutrophils are often a part of a mixed inflammatory infiltrate (Figure 1-1).
■ Distended or ruptured glands can be denuded of epithelium containing abundant debris and neutrophils (Figure 1-2), and may form an abscess (Figure 1-3).

(text continued on page 4)

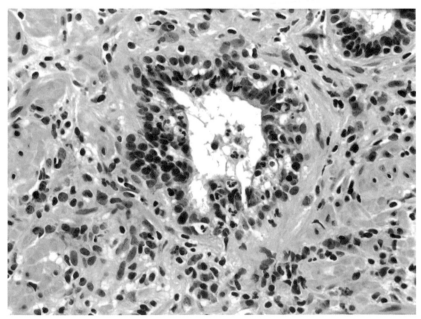

FIGURE 1-1

FIGURE 1-1   Luminal, intraepithelial, and stromal acute inflammation accompanied by a mixed inflammatory infiltrate of lymphocytes and histiocytes. The gland demonstrates atrophy.

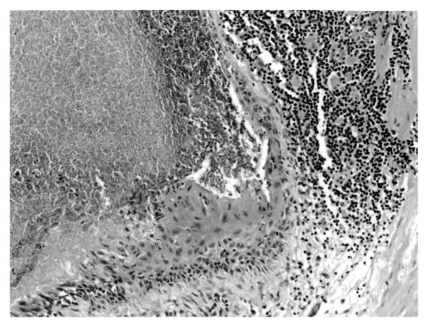

FIGURE 1-2

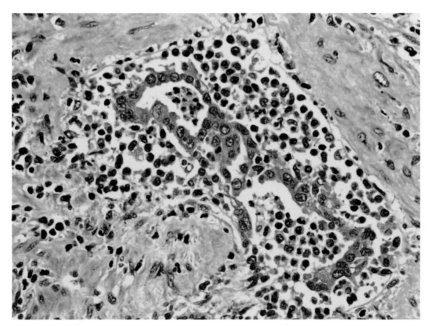

FIGURE 1-3

FIGURE 1-2   Dilated gland filled with debris and acute inflammation is seen with adjacent lymphocytic inflammation.

FIGURE 1-3   Abscess formation with soughed remaining glandular epithelium admixed with the acute and chronic inflammatory infiltrate.

Acute Inflammation (*continued*)

- Neutrophilic infiltrates may be associated with nuclear atypia, including increased nucleolar prominence.
- Acute inflammation is associated with a variety of nonneoplastic epithelial alterations, including atrophy, hyperplasia, squamous metaplasia, and transitional metaplasia.

ANCILLARY STUDIES
- Gram stain may be utilized if abscess formation is seen in an immunocompromised patient but ancillary testing is not necessary in immunocompetent patients.
- Basal cell markers, including p63 and high molecular weight keratin (HMWK), can aid in the discrimination of nuclear atypia due to acute inflammation and prostatic adenocarcinoma.

DIFFERENTIAL DIAGNOSIS
- Prostatic adenocarcinoma (atrophic type) and high-grade prostatic intraepithelial neoplasia: The nucleolar prominence in neoplastic prostatic glands is more marked than that associated with acute inflammation, which tends to have pinpoint nucleoli. Prostatic adenocarcinoma has an infiltrative growth pattern lacking basal cells while high-grade prostatic intraepithelial neoplasia demonstrates a greater degree of cellular stratification and gland complexity. Additionally, acute inflammation is only rarely present in neoplastic prostate glands (Figure 1-4).

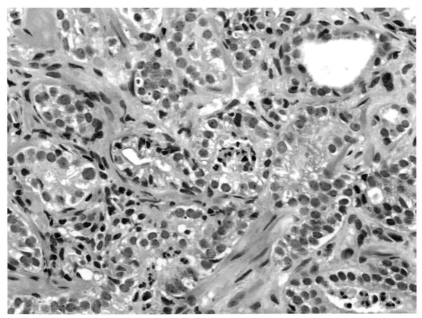

FIGURE 1-4

FIGURE 1-4   Prostatic adenocarcinoma with abundant intraluminal inflammation, a rare finding. Note nucleomegaly and macronucleoli not seen in nonneoplastic glands.

Chronic Inflammation

DEFINITION
- Lymphoplasmacytic infiltrate involving the prostate.

CLINICAL FEATURES
- Typically chronic inflammation is not associated with the presence of organisms and may be due to obstruction or iatrogenic causes.
- The contribution of abundant chronic inflammation to serum PSA elevation is controversial.
- Chronic inflammation within the prostate is nearly ubiquitous and does not need to be mentioned in a pathology report unless the infiltrate is marked.
- The term "chronic prostatitis" should be avoided as prostatitis implies clinical sequelae.

MICROSCOPIC FEATURES
- Lymphoplasmacytic infiltrate is usually periglandular (Figure 1-5) or stromal (Figure 1-6), with or without other types of inflammatory cells.
- Epithelial alterations, including atrophy and squamous or transitional metaplasia, may accompany the chronic inflammation (Figure 1-7).
- Lymphocytes may show perinuclear clearing, giving the appearance of signet ring cells (Figure 1-8).

ANCILLARY STUDIES
- CD3 and CD20 may be utilized to demonstrate a mixture of T and B lymphocytes if lymphoma is a diagnostic consideration.
- CD45 can be used to highlight the lymphocytes. A lack of expression using a broad spectrum cytokeratin (AE1/3, CAM5.2 or pancytokeratin) in addition to negativity using a prostate-specific marker such as PSA or prostate-specific acid phosphatase (PSAP) can be utilized to rule out high-grade prostatic adenocarcinoma and lack of synaptophysin and chromogranin can rule out small cell carcinoma.

DIFFERENTIAL DIAGNOSIS
- Lymphoma: Monotonous, diffuse infiltrates raise the differential diagnosis of lymphoma while mixed infiltrates favor nonneoplastic chronic inflammation.
- High-grade prostatic adenocarcinoma: Gleason pattern 5 prostatic adenocarcinoma may have an appearance similar to cords or sheets of lymphocytes with signet ring cell change. Careful inspection of the cells and identification of lower grade areas of tumor with glandular differentiation can be helpful.
- Small cell carcinoma: Small cell carcinoma is composed of cells that are larger than a lymphocyte, with a higher mitotic rate, and abundant karyorrhectic bodies.

(continued)

Chronic Inflammation (continued)

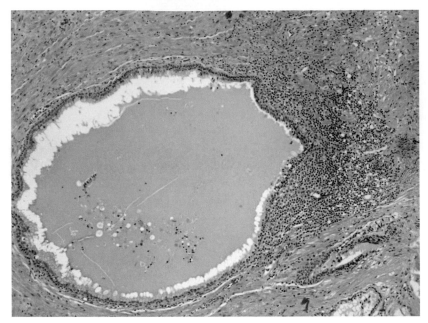

FIGURE 1-5

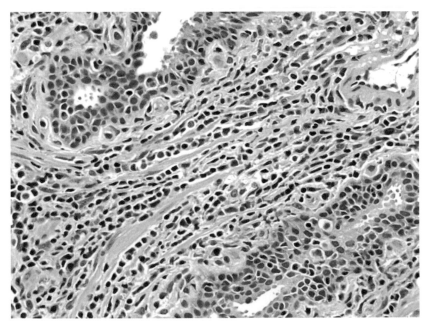

FIGURE 1-6

FIGURE 1-5 Periglandular lymphocytic infiltration surrounding a dilated gland.

FIGURE 1-6 A stromal infiltrate of lymphocytes is present.

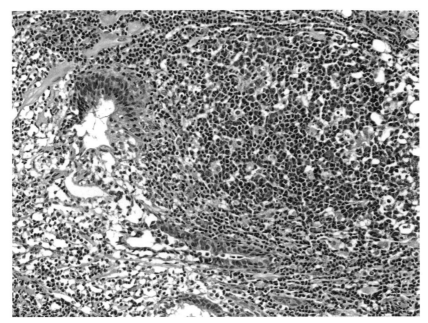

FIGURE 1-7

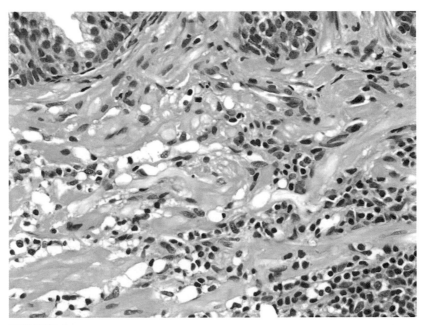

FIGURE 1-8

FIGURE 1-7   Abundant chronic inflammation with follicle formation is present admixed with atrophic prostatic glands.

FIGURE 1-8   Signet ring and clear cell change due to thermal artifact is seen within lymphocytes. This can mimic high-grade prostatic adenocarcinoma.

Granulomatous Inflammation

DEFINITION
■ Granulomatous inflammation involving the prostate due to nonspecific causes, post-procedures, infectious agents or systemic disease that may result in PSA elevation.

CLINICAL FEATURES
■ Nonspecific granulomatous reaction is due to blocked prostatic ducts/acini and is the most common form of granulomatous prostatitis.
■ Post-procedural granulomatous reaction is the second most common cause of granulomatous inflammation within the prostate and may be seen following transurethral resections or needle core biopsies.
■ Bacillus Calmette-Guerin (BCG)-related therapy, bacterial, fungal, parasitic, and viral pathogens may result in granulomatous inflammation.
■ The term "granulomatous prostatitis" should be avoided as prostatitis implies clinical sequelae.

MICROSCOPIC FEATURES
■ Nonspecific granulomatous prostatitis is composed of ducts and acini filled with sloughed epithelium and a mixed inflammatory infiltrate with extension into the surrounding stroma (Figure 1-9).
■ Post-procedural tissue may show well-formed granuloma demonstrating a central region of coagulative necrosis circumscribed by palisading histiocytes and foreign body giant cells.
■ BCG-related therapy and other pathogens can produce well-formed caseating and noncaseating granulomata or diffuse granulomatous inflammation (Figure 1-10).

(text continued on page 10)

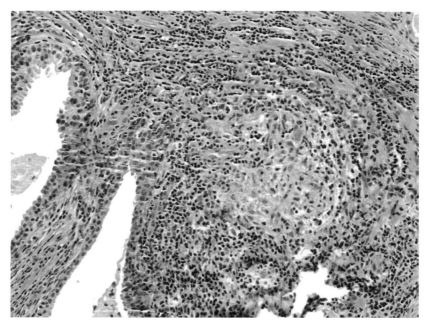

FIGURE 1-9

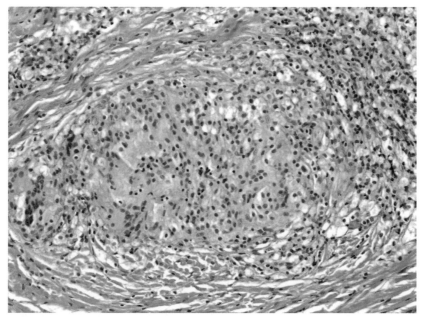

FIGURE 1-10

FIGURE 1-9   Nonspecific granulomatous inflammation is seen adjacent to atrophic glands and lymphoplasmacytic inflammation.

FIGURE 1-10   Granuloma post-BCG treatment.

Granulomatous Inflammation *(continued)*

ANCILLARY STUDIES
- Positivity for CD68 and CD163 along with no expression using a broad spectrum cytokeratin (AE1/3, CAM5.2 or pancytokeratin) can be used to confirm the histiocytic nature of the infiltrate (Figures 1-11 and 1-12).
- For immunocompromised patients or those suspected to have systemic infections, periodic acid-Schiff (PAS), Gomori methenamine silver (GMS), and acid fast bacillus (AFB) stains may be performed.
- Calcium and iron stains can be used if malakoplakia is a consideration.

DIFFERENTIAL DIAGNOSIS
- Post-therapy prostatic adenocarcinoma: Prostatic adenocarcinoma post-treatment with gonadotropin-releasing hormone (GnRH) analogs, such as leuprolide, and other chemotherapeutic agents may show single cells, foamy cytoplasm, and less nucleolar prominence, thus mimicking histiocytes. Identifying residual glands, using immunohistochemistry, and the clinical context can differentiate these entities.
- High-grade prostatic adenocarcinoma: Diffuse sheets and single cells of Gleason pattern 5 prostatic adenocarcinoma may mimic granulomatous inflammation. Nucleolar prominence is typically more pronounced.
- Malakoplakia: Defective phagolysosomes give rise to large histiocytes (von Hansemann cells) containing laminated calcium phosphate crystals (Michaelis–Gutmann bodies).

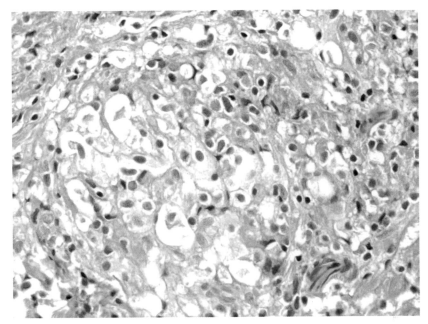

FIGURE 1-11

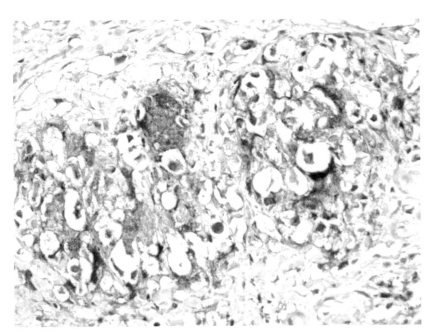

FIGURE 1-12

FIGURE 1-11   Diffuse granulomatous inflammation may mimic post-therapy or high-grade prostatic adenocarcinoma.

FIGURE 1-12   Expression with CD68 in the cells shown in Figure 1-11 confirms that the infiltrate is granulomatous inflammation.

ATROPHY

Atrophy Overview

DEFINITION
■ Decreased cytoplasmic volume of nonneoplastic prostatic acinar luminal cells.

CLINICAL FEATURES
■ Associated with an increase in serum PSA, with extent of atrophy purported to correlate with the amount of PSA elevation.
■ Occurs in conjunction with acute and/or chronic prostatitis.
■ Increases in incidence with age and is present in virtually all middle-aged men but is not associated with prostate gland volume.
■ Most frequently occurs in the peripheral zone.
■ Hypothesized to be an injury response caused by chronic ischemia due to locoregional arteriosclerosis and may also be induced by radiation treatment or androgen ablation.
■ Atrophy has minimal to no association with an increase in finding carcinoma or high-grade prostatic intraepithelial neoplasia on subsequent biopsy.
■ Identifying atrophy is important to avoid confusion with neoplastic entities.
■ A variety of classification schemes have been proposed based on the degree of glandular atrophy and surrounding stomal changes, including the following: partial, simple, simple with cyst formation, sclerotic, postatrophic hyperplasia (or hyperplastic), and proliferative inflammatory.
■ As there is no impact on patient care based on the presence of atrophy, it is not necessary for the pathologist to comment on its presence, type, or extent.

MICROSCOPIC FEATURES
■ A decrease in the volume of cytoplasm is seen, yielding an increase in nuclear to cytoplasmic ratio. The decrease in cytoplasm can be moderate, invoking minimal microscopic changes, with cells retaining pale eosinophilic cytoplasm (Figure 1-13), to severe, with glands having a basophilic, flattened and dilated appearance (Figure 1-14).

(text continued on page 14)

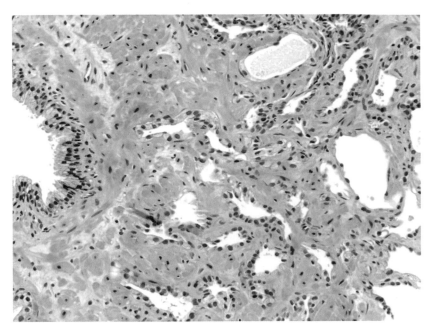

FIGURE 1-13

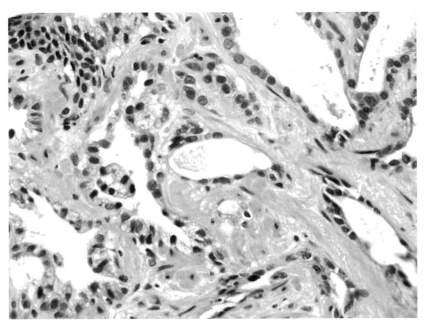

FIGURE 1-14

FIGURE 1-13   Haphazard infiltrative atrophic glands are seen with a variable decrease in cytoplasm, ranging from partially atrophic to complete atrophy. A single nonatrophic gland is present in the left side of the photomicrograph.

FIGURE 1-14   Atrophic angular basophilic glands demonstrate straight luminal borders, flattened epithelium, dilated lumina, and cytoplasmic membranes abutting the nuclei.

Chapter 1: Nonneoplastic Conditions   *13*

Atrophy Overview *(continued)*

ANCILLARY STUDIES
- Basal cell markers, including p63 and HMWK, can help differentiate atrophy from adenocarcinoma. However, basal cell markers can demonstrate patchy positivity and occasional glands may be negative (Figure 1-15). Additionally, alpha-methylacyl-CoA racemase (AMACR) can be weakly positive.

DIFFERENTIAL DIAGNOSIS
- Prostatic adenocarcinoma (atrophic type): Adenocarcinoma is infiltrative while atrophy more often has a lobular pattern. Adenocarcinoma will have more cytoplasm and atrophy will have less, which can impart a basophilic appearance with nuclei nearly touching the cytoplasmic membrane. Nuclear and nucleolar prominence are more pronounced in adenocarcinoma (Figure 1-16). Atrophy is more frequently associated with inflammation (luminal, transepithelial, and periglandular).
- High-grade prostatic intraepithelial neoplasia: High-grade prostatic intraepithelial neoplasia can appear similar to atrophy. However, high-grade prostatic intraepithelial neoplasia will have nuclear stratification and a degree of nucleomegaly not seen in atrophy.
- Basal cell hyperplasia: Basal cell hyperplasia imparts a basophilic appearance to glands and has scant cytoplasm, but unlike atrophy, is multilayered and has nuclei that are more crowded and overlapping.

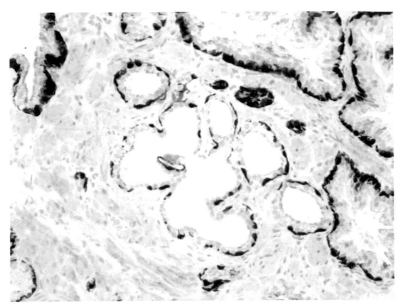

FIGURE 1-15

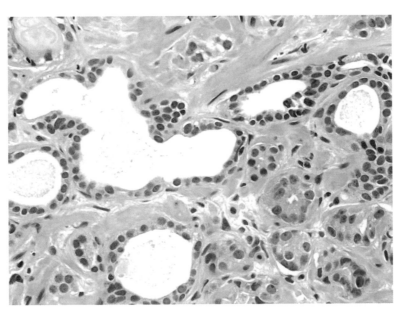

FIGURE 1-16

FIGURE 1-15   A triple immunostain of p63 (brown), HMWK (brown), and AMACR (pink) reveal
patching basal cells in atrophic glands in the center of the photomicrograph in comparison
to adjacent nonatrophic glands with a much more prominent, continuous basal cell layer.

FIGURE 1-16   Dilated, atrophic glands are adjacent to well-differentiated prostatic adenocarcinoma,
seen in the lower right corner. Atrophic glands have pinpoint nucleoli in comparison
to the macronucleoli of adenocarcinoma. Note that the cell membrane appears to lie on
top of the atrophic nuclei in contrast to the malignant glands that have an observable
space between the cell membrane and nuclei.

Partial Atrophy

DEFINITION
- Partial loss of cytoplasm resulting in pale, eosinophilic disorganized nonneoplastic glands that can mimic prostatic adenocarcinoma.

CLINICAL FEATURES
- No association with increased risk of prostatic adenocarcinoma or high-grade prostatic intraepithelial neoplasia.
- Partial atrophy versus prostatic adenocarcinoma is the diagnostic dilemma most often prompting a consultation in a prostate needle biopsy.

MICROSCOPIC FEATURES
- Crowded glands with a disorganized growth pattern (Figure 1-17).
- Glands show a range of luminal shapes, including infoldings, undulations, as well as areas with straight luminal borders (Figure 1-18).
- The cytoplasm is decreased but is visible as pale and eosinophilic.
- Usually stroma separates the glands, with only occasional back-to-back glands.
- Mild nuclear and nucleolar enlargement. Occasional nuclei appear to touch the cytoplasmic membrane.
- Basal cells are difficult to identify.

(text continued on page 18)

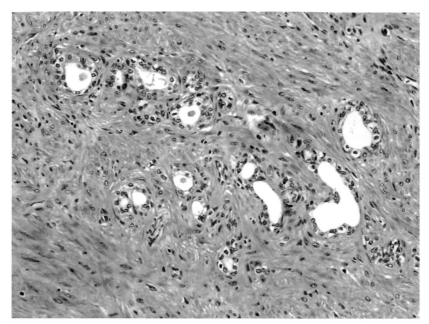

FIGURE 1-17

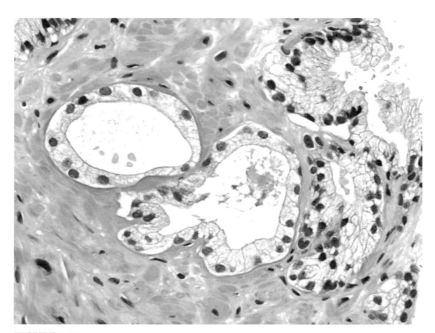

FIGURE 1-18

FIGURE 1-17   A lobule of partial atrophic glands with a crowded, infiltrative appearance.

FIGURE 1-18   Straight and infolded luminal contours are seen in these partially atrophic glands. The decrease in cytoplasm is evident when compared to the nonatrophic glands on the right.

Partial Atrophy *(continued)*

ANCILLARY STUDIES
- Basal cell markers, such as p63 and HMWK, show decreased, patchy expression and AMACR can be weakly positive (Figures 1-19 and 1-20).

DIFFERENTIAL DIAGNOSIS
- Prostatic adenocarcinoma: Adenocarcinoma is the main differential diagnosis of partial atrophy. While partial atrophy has slight nuclear and nucleolar prominence, it is not to the degree seen in well-differentiated prostatic adenocarcinoma. Additionally, adenocarcinoma has a more consistently straight luminal border. Importantly, the expression pattern of basal cell markers and AMACR overlap between partial atrophy and adenocarcinoma.

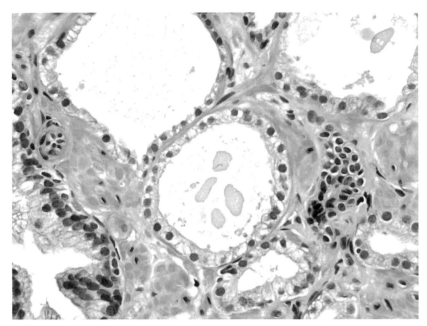

FIGURE 1-19

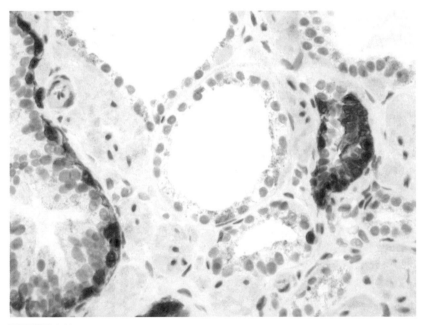

FIGURE 1-20

FIGURE 1-19 Partially atrophic glands are nearly back-to-back, with minimal pale, eosinophilic cytoplasm remaining.

FIGURE 1-20 A triple immunostain of p63 (brown), HMWK (brown), and AMACR (pink) of the photomicrograph in Figure 1-19. Note that only rare basal cells are detected in the atrophic glands and that AMACR shows weak reactivity. Adjacent nonatrophic glands are present.

Other Types of Atrophy

DEFINITION
- Decrease in cytoplasmic volume of prostatic luminal cells imparting a basophilic appearance.

CLINICAL FEATURES
- Conflicting studies regarding an association with a minimal increased risk in prostatic adenocarcinoma.
- A variety of categories have been proposed to classify types of atrophy in addition to the category of partial atrophy. These categories represent a continuum and are typically present in multiple forms within the same specimen. It is not necessary to acknowledge the presence of atrophy in a pathology report or to attempt to identify the subtype.

MICROSCOPIC FEATURES
- Simple atrophy involves most to all of a lobule (Figure 1-21) with small acini that have a round to angular shape, flattened, cuboidal epithelium, and scant cytoplasm imparting a basophilic low-power appearance (Figure 1-22). The cell membrane lies against the nucleus, yielding a high nuclear to cytoplasmic ratio. Luminal corpora amylacea, stromal sclerosis, and acute and chronic inflammation may be present.
- Dilated glands of simple atrophy are termed simple atrophy with cyst formation.

(text continued on page 22)

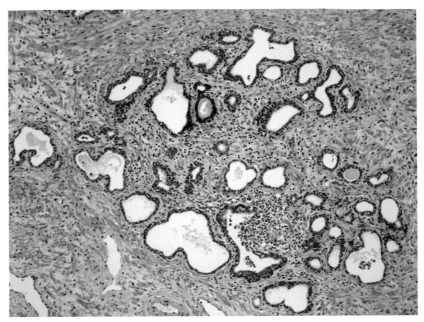

FIGURE 1-21

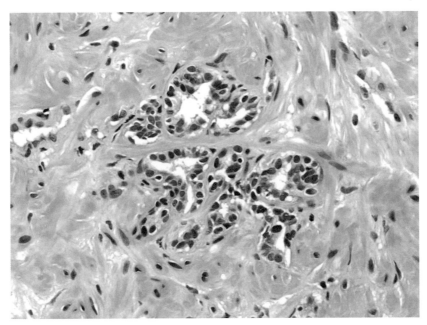

FIGURE 1-22

FIGURE 1-21   A lobule is involved by simple and cystic atrophy, with a basophilic appearance at low power.

FIGURE 1-22   Simple atrophy at high magnification reveals darkly staining nuclei and minimal cytoplasm.

Other Types of Atrophy (*continued*)

- Sclerotic atrophy demonstrates marked sclerosis surrounding the acini, producing angular, distorted glands that have an infiltrative appearance (Figure 1-23).
- Postatrophic hyperplasia (hyperplastic atrophy) has a central dilated duct with surrounding smaller atrophic acini in a lobular configuration (Figure 1-24).
- Proliferative inflammatory atrophy has an inflammatory infiltrate and an increased mitotic rate, overlapping with the previously mentioned categories.

ANCILLARY STUDIES
- The basal cell markers, p63 and HMWK, are typically positive while AMACR is usually negative.

DIFFERENTIAL DIAGNOSIS
- Prostatic adenocarcinoma (atrophic type): Adenocarcinoma can mimic simple and sclerotic atrophy. Searching for areas of classic adenocarcinoma and use of immunohistochemistry will resolve this differential.
- High-grade prostatic intraepithelial neoplasia: This is a diagnostic consideration with simple and sclerotic atrophy due to the basophilic appearance, but is differentiated due to the nuclear stratification and the presence of nucleoli at 20x magnification.
- Basal cell hyperplasia: Basal cell hyperplasia can be confused with simple atrophy due to the basophilic appearance, although basal cell hyperplasia will have multiple layers and more pronounced nuclear overlap.

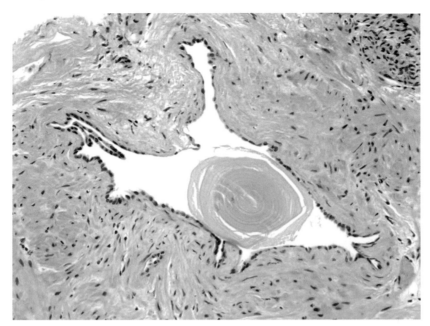

FIGURE 1-23

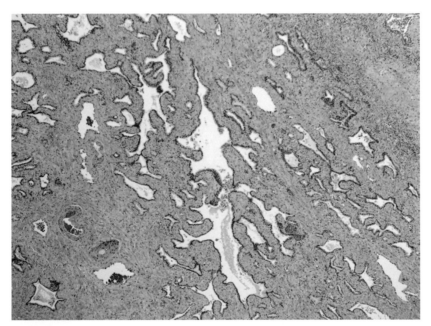

FIGURE 1-24

FIGURE 1-23 Sclerotic atrophy results in unusual, infiltrative appearing glandular shapes. The presence of intraluminal corpora amylacea is consistent with the nonneoplastic nature of atrophy.

FIGURE 1-24 A central dilated gland surrounded by atrophic smaller glands is characteristic of postatrophic hyperplasia.

ADENOSIS

DEFINITION
■ Crowded nonneoplastic prostatic glands mimicking low-grade prostatic adenocarcinoma.

CLINICAL FEATURES
■ Incidental histiologic finding that is more common in the transition zone and more frequently seen in transurethral resection specimens than needle core biopsies.
■ Patients are not at increased risk for having prostatic adenocarcinoma. Adenosis is only clinically relevant in that it must be distinguished from carcinoma. It is not necessary to acknowledge the presence of adenosis in a pathology report.

MICROSCOPIC FEATURES
■ Nodular, well-circumscribed proliferation of small, crowded glands (Figure 1-25).
■ Glands have pale cytoplasm and predominantly bland nuclei lacking prominent nucleoli (Figure 1-26).

(text continued on page 26)

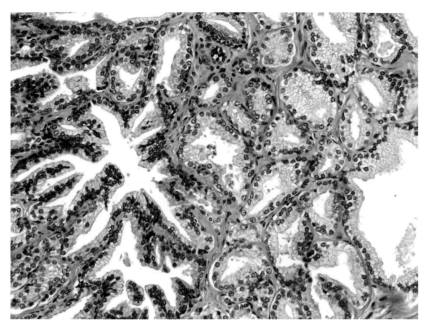

FIGURE 1-25

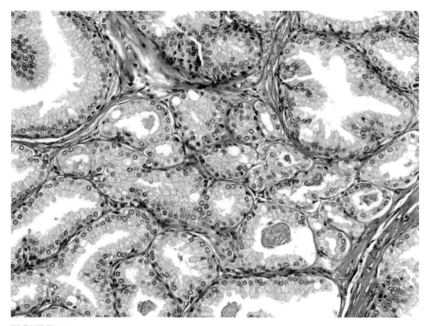

FIGURE 1-26

FIGURE 1-25 Adenosis with small crowded glands is seen, admixed with glands with undulating cell membranes, typical of nonneoplastic prostatic glands.

FIGURE 1-26 The glands of adenosis have pale, abundant cytoplasm with bland nuclei.

Adenosis *(continued)*

- Flattened basal cells circumscribe the glands but may be difficult to visualize (Figure 1-27).
- Occasional larger glands with an undulating apical membrane are present.

ANCILLARY STUDIES
- Basal cell markers, such as p63 and HMWK, show patchy reactivity while AMACR has variable expression.

DIFFERENTIAL DIAGNOSIS
- Low-grade prostatic adenocarcinoma: Adenocarcinoma can be confused with adenosis although it has a more infiltrative growth pattern and more frequent macronucleoli (Figure 1-28). Occasional larger, more classic appearing nonneoplastic glands intermixed with adenosis can help differentiate adenosis from carcinoma. Additionally, immunostains may help appreciate basal cells in adenosis although AMACR expression demonstrates overlap between adenosis and carcinoma.

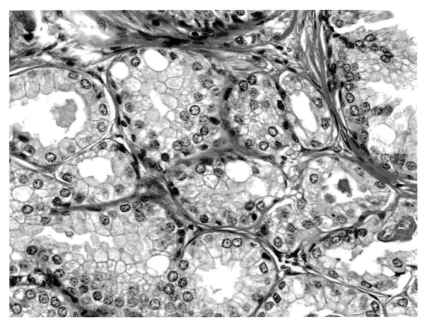

FIGURE 1-27

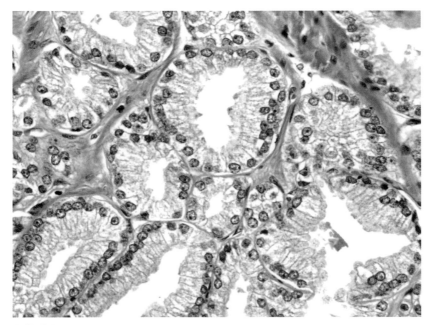

FIGURE 1-28

FIGURE 1-27   Flattened basal cells are seen at high power in this focus of adenosis. Only pinpoint nucleoli are evident.

FIGURE 1-28   This low-grade prostatic adenocarcinoma has small crowded glands similar to adenosis, but has readily apparent macronucleoli.

HYPERPLASIA

Benign Prostatic Hyperplasia

DEFINITION
■ Nonneoplastic increase in number of prostatic epithelial and stromal cells.

CLINICAL FEATURES
■ Most common urologic condition in men.
■ Increases with age and is present in the majority of elderly men.
■ Periurethral location is frequent.
■ Nodules compress the urethra and cause urinary obstruction with symptoms such as increased urinary frequency, hesitation, dribbling, and incomplete bladder emptying.
■ Most common cause of serum prostate-specific antigen elevation.
■ Diagnosed based on clinical findings and the histologic presence of nodules, therefore, is diagnosed in transurethral specimens and not needle core biopsies.

MICROSCOPIC FEATURES
■ Nodules composed of varying amounts of glands (Figure 1-29) and stroma (Figure 1-30).
■ Stromal only nodules may be seen and are composed of fibromuscular cells, occasional small blood vessels, and scattered chronic inflammation. The stroma may be myxoid or hyalinized (Figure 1-31).
■ Glands appear unremarkable, with a nondescript acinar and basal cell layer, or may have papillary infoldings (Figure 1-32).

ANCILLARY STUDIES
■ None.

DIFFERENTIAL DIAGNOSIS
■ Stromal tumor of uncertain malignant potential: Benign prostatic hyperplasia may mimic these tumors but lack the stromal atypia and sheet-like stroma without nodule formation seen in stromal tumor of uncertain malignant potential.

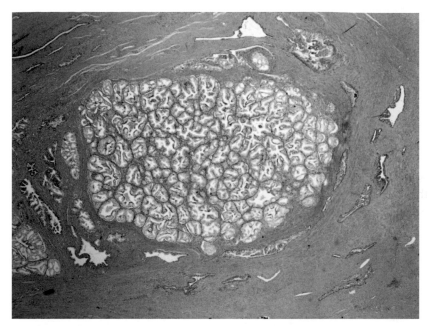

FIGURE 1-29

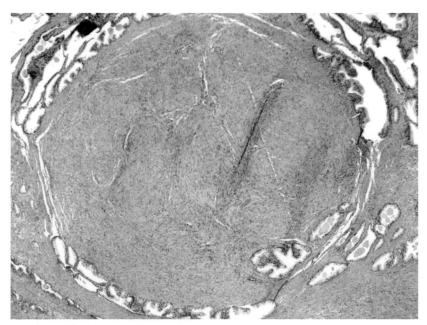

FIGURE 1-30

(continued)

FIGURE 1-29   Some nodules contain mostly prostatic glands with minimal stroma.

FIGURE 1-30   This nodule is composed of mostly stroma with compressed glands at the periphery.

Benign Prostatic Hyperplasia (*continued*)

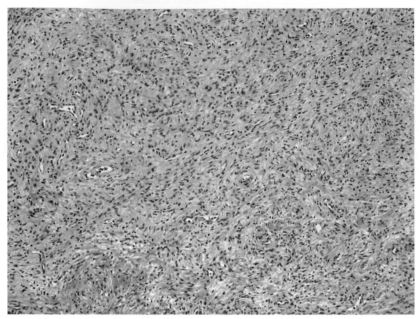

FIGURE 1-31

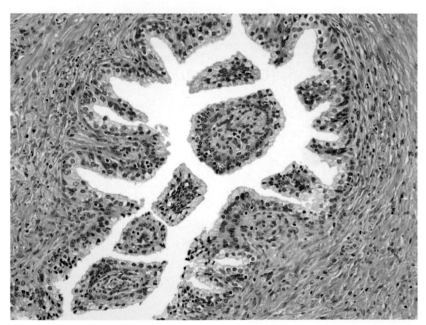

FIGURE 1-32

FIGURE 1-31　Bland fibromuscular spindle cells with small blood vessels and a slightly myxoid stroma form this stromal nodule.

FIGURE 1-32　Glands appear bland and can have papillary infoldings, which on cross section appear as fibrovascular cores floating within the lumen.

Basal Cell Hyperplasia

DEFINITION
- Glandular proliferation composed of basophilic cells with a basaloid phenotype.

CLINICAL FEATURES
- More common in the transition zone.
- May be associated with antiandrogen therapy.

MICROSCOPIC FEATURES
- Nodular proliferation of small glands composed of cells with multiple layers of basal cells and minimal cytoplasm, conferring a basophilic appearance (Figure 1-33).
- Eosinophilic intraluminal secretions are often present.

(text continued on page 32)

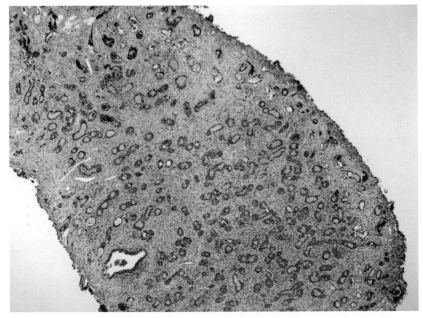

FIGURE 1-33

FIGURE 1-33 This nodule of basal cell hyperplasia was identified in the transition zone from a transurethral resection. Note that the glands are uniformly spaced apart.

Basal Cell Hyperplasia (*continued*)

■ Nuclei are crowded and bland, lacking macronucleoli (Figure 1-34).
■ Cribriform architecture, intraluminal calcification, intracytoplasmic hyaline globules, and squamous metaplasia may be seen (Figure 1-35).

ANCILLARY STUDIES
■ Basal cell markers will be positive, with p63 described as having more reliable positivity than HMWK, particularly in the transition zone. AMACR is negative.

DIFFERENTIAL DIAGNOSIS
■ Prostatic adenocarcinoma: Adenocarcinoma may be confused with basal cell hyperplasia due to the small glands, occasional cribriform formation, and rare infiltrative growth (Figure 1-36). However, bland nuclei and lack of macronuclei aid in excluding carcinoma. Immunostains can differentiate the entities, with the use of multiple basal cell markers recommended as HMWK may be negative in both cancer and basal cell hyperplasia.
■ High-grade prostatic intraepithelial neoplasia: High-grade prostatic intraepithelial neoplasia may have a basophilic appearance and complex architecture, although macronuclei will be visualized and a well-circumscribed appearance will not be seen.
■ Basal cell carcinoma: Basal cell carcinoma is a basaloid lesion that shows extensive infiltrative into nonneoplastic glands, can have necrosis, perineural invasion, multiple growth patterns, and a high proliferation rate.

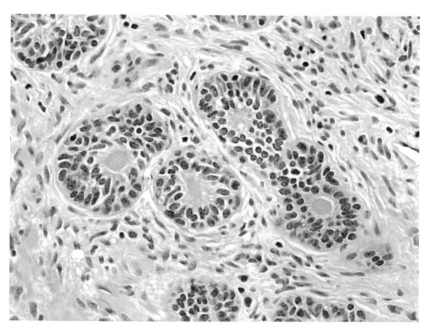

FIGURE 1-34

FIGURE 1-34   At high power, basal cell hyperplasia reveals basal cells which are oriented both parallel and perpendicular to the basement membrane, have bland, crowded nuclei with pinpoint nucleoli, and minimal cytoplasm.

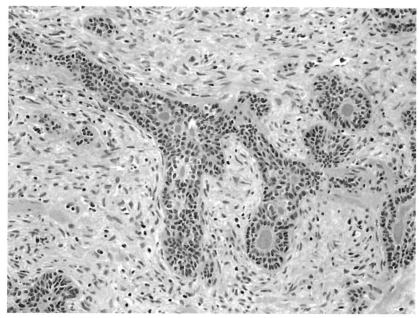

FIGURE 1-35

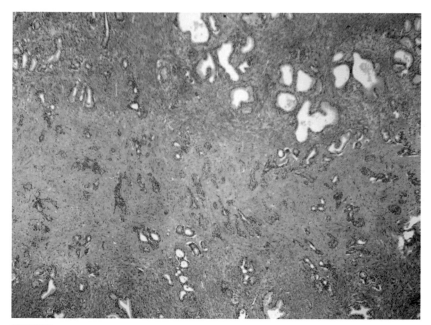

FIGURE 1-36

FIGURE 1-35   A cribriform/pseudocribriform space is seen within this gland of basal cell hyperplasia.

FIGURE 1-36   Basal cell hyperplasia in this prostatectomy specimen has formed in a scar, giving an infiltrative appearance that mimics adenocarcinoma.

Clear Cell Cribriform Hyperplasia

DEFINITION
- Nonneoplastic hyperplastic cribriform prostatic glands with pale cytoplasm.

CLINICAL FEATURES
- Uncommon form of benign prostatic hyperplasia.
- Usually located in the transition zone.
- More typically encountered in transurethral resection specimens than needle core biopsies.
- No clinical significance.

MICROSCOPIC FEATURES
- Crowed glands with interspersed or nodular growth (Figure 1-37).
- Glands are cribriformed with lumens of varying sizes (Figure 1-38).

(text continued on page 36)

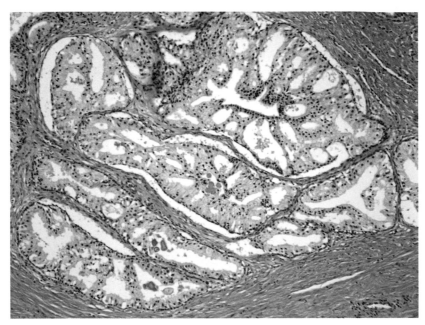

FIGURE 1-37

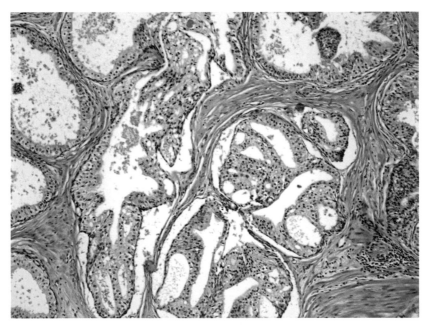

FIGURE 1-38

FIGURE 1-37   Glands of clear cell cribriform hyperplasia grow close together.

FIGURE 1-38   Cribriform spaces vary in size and shape.

Clear Cell Cribriform Hyperplasia *(continued)*

■ Basal cells surround the glands (Figure 1-39).
■ Nuclei are bland, uniform, and small in size, and lack prominent nucleoli (Figure 1-40).

ANCILLARY STUDIES
■ Basal cell markers, such as p63 and HMWK, will highlight basal cells in clear cell cribriform hyperplasia. AMACR is weak to negative.

DIFFERENTIAL DIAGNOSIS
■ High-grade prostatic intraepithelial neoplasia: Clear cell cribriform hyperplasia lacks prominent nucleoli unlike high-grade prostatic intraepithelial neoplasia. The cytoplasm of high-grade prostatic intraepithelial neoplasia is denser and more chromophilic.
■ Prostatic adenocarcinoma, Gleason pattern 4: Gleason pattern 4 prostatic adenocarcinoma can have a cribriform pattern. However, unlike clear cell cribriform hyperplasia, nucleomegaly and prominent nucleoli will be present and basal cells will be absent.
■ Prostatic adenocarcinoma, foamy variant: Both foamy variant of prostatic adenocarcinoma and clear cell cribriform hyperplasia can have pale cytoplasm and bland nuclei. Foamy variant of prostatic adenocarcinoma typically does not show hyperplastic glands or cribriform architecture, and lacks basal cells.

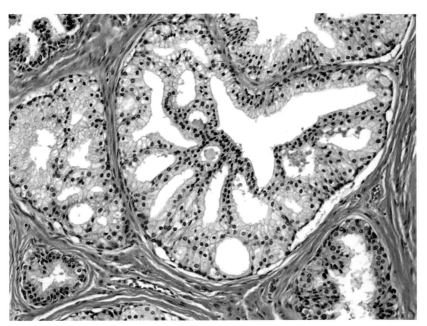

FIGURE 1-39

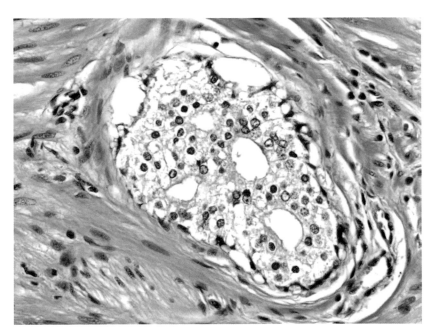

FIGURE 1-40

FIGURE 1-39   Basal cells are seen surrounding glands of clear cell cribriform hyperplasia.

FIGURE 1-40   Nuclei are small with only pinpoint nucleoli present.

METAPLASIA

Transitional and Squamous Cell Metaplasia

DEFINITION
■ Transitional (urothelial) or squamous cells lining prostatic ducts or glands.

CLINICAL FEATURES
■ Frequent incidental finding.
■ Difficult to discern if the process represents normal anatomical variation or a pathologic process.
■ May be induced by tissue damage as has been associated with inflammation, infarction, and post therapy.

MICROSCOPIC FEATURES
■ Transitional cell metaplasia is seen in glands typically near the urethra. Glands may show a spectrum of changes similar to that in the bladder, including von Brunn's nests and cystitis cystica with punched out lumens (Figure 1-41). The glands have a basophilic appearance populated with cells that are columnar and stream in an orientation perpendicular to the basement membrane. The cytoplasm is minimal and pale. Perinuclear clearing and nuclear grooves are present (Figure 1-42).
■ Squamous cell metaplasia is found in crowded glands with small lumens, often accompanied by inflammation. Intercellular bridges and dense eosinophilic cytoplasm are seen (Figure 1-43). Radiation and hormone therapy leads to immature squamous metaplasia with cells having less abundant cytoplasm that can have atypical nuclei. Keratin pearls are uncommon.

(text continued on page 40)

FIGURE 1-41 This focus of transitional cell metaplasia shows a characteristic clover-like arrangement and punched out lumina filled with eosinophilic material.

FIGURE 1-42 A portion of residual normal prostatic gland is seen in the upper left-hand corner while the rest of the gland is filled with transitional cell metaplasia. The cells stream toward the luminal space. Nuclear clearing is seen.

FIGURE 1-43 This gland has a protrusion of cells with squamous cell metaplasia, showing pronounced intercellular bridges and bright eosinophilic cytoplasm.

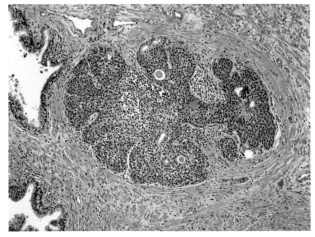

FIGURE 1-41

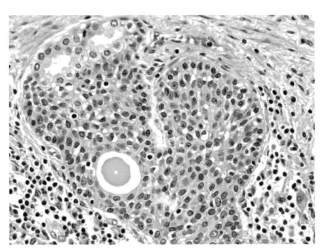

FIGURE 1-42

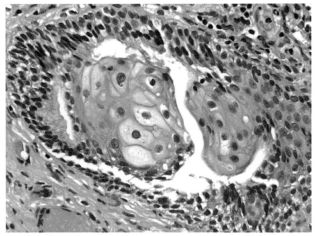

FIGURE 1-43

Transitional and Squamous Cell Metaplasia (*continued*)

ANCILLARY STUDIES
- Basal cell markers (p63 and HMWK) will highlight metaplastic cells. PSA and PSAP have variable reactivity. Ki-67 is low.

DIFFERENTIAL DIAGNOSIS
- High-grade prostatic intraepithelial neoplasia: Transitional and squamous cell metaplasia can mimic high-grade prostatic intraepithelial neoplasia, although high-grade prostatic intraepithelial neoplasia will have nucleolar prominence not found in metaplasia (Figure 1-44).
- Squamous cell carcinoma: Squamous cell carcinoma of the prostate is extremely rare. In contrast to squamous cell metaplasia, carcinoma will have marked nuclear hyperchromasia and atypia and abnormal mitotic figures. It also will not show a geographic association with areas of infarctions or inflammation.

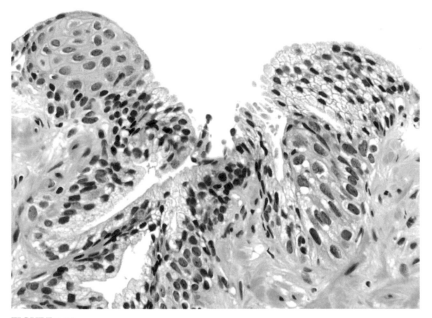

FIGURE 1-44

FIGURE 1-44   In this needle core biopsy, a prostate gland contains two foci of squamous cell metaplasia (upper left and right side). Although there is nucleomegaly, this should not be construed as high-grade prostatic intraepithelial neoplasia. Note the absence of prominent nuceoli.

DEFINITION
- Nonneoplastic prostate glands with mucin-filled apical cells.

CLINICAL FEATURES
- Incidental finding with no clinical significance other than histologic recognition to prevent incorrect interpretation.

MICROSCOPIC FEATURES
- Clusters of glands that may form a lobule with columnar acinar cells containing abundant clear to blue cytoplasm (Figures 1-45 and 1-46).
- Mucinous metaplasia can be associated with atrophy, other types of metaplasia, and hyperplasia (Figure 1-47).
- Nuclei are small and round to flattened. As the acinar cell nuclei are pushed towards the basal surface, basal cells may be difficult to visualize without immunohistochemistry (Figure 1-48).

ANCILLARY STUDIES
- Basal cell markers (p63 and HMWK) will highlight basal cells. PSA and PSAP are negative.

DIFFERENTIAL DIAGNOSIS
- Prostatic adenocarcinoma: Mucinous metaplasia can be mistaken for classic well-differentiated prostatic adenocarcinoma or foamy variant. In contrast to mucinous metaplasia, classic prostatic adenocarcinoma will have nucleomegaly and prominent nucleoli. Both classic prostatic adenocarcinoma and foamy variant will lack expression with basal cell markers and will be positive for AMACR, PSA, and PSAP.
- Cowper's glands: This structure may be admixed with skeletal muscle and will not have surrounding unremarkable prostatic glands.

(continued)

Mucinous Metaplasia (*continued*)

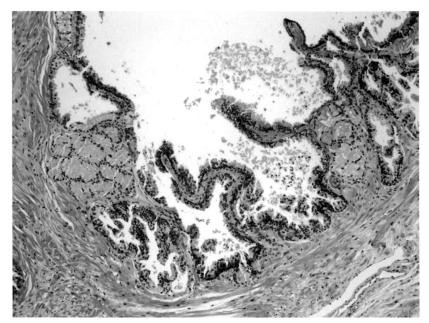

FIGURE 1-45

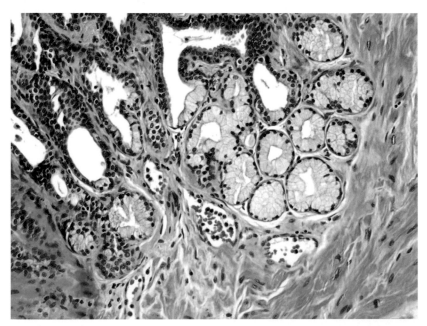

FIGURE 1-46

FIGURE 1-45   Clusters of glands demonstrating mucinous metaplasia are seen with admixed nonmetaplastic glands.

FIGURE 1-46   Mucinous metaplasia is usually a small lesion and may only partially involve prostatic glands and ducts.

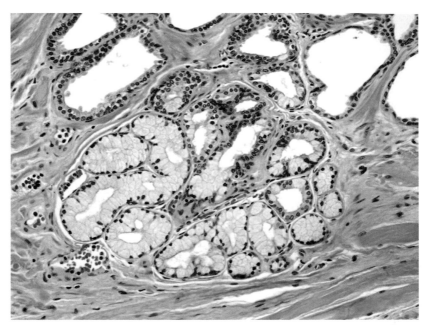

FIGURE 1-47

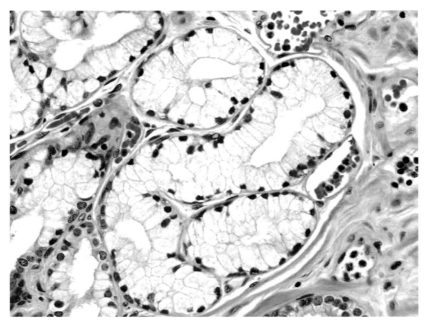

FIGURE 1-48

FIGURE 1-47   Atrophy may be seen adjacent to areas of mucinous metaplasia.

FIGURE 1-48   At high magnification, bland hyperchromatic nuclei appear flattened by mucin-filled goblet cells and basal cells are difficult to visualize.

Chapter 1: Nonneoplastic Conditions   43

Nephrogenic Metaplasia

DEFINITION
■ Small glands with renal tubular expression occurring along the urothelial tract.

CLINICAL FEATURES
■ This is an incidental finding associated with prior urothelial trauma or renal transplantation.
■ The etiology of the lesion may be from displaced renal tubular cells.
■ It is important to recognize this lesion to prevent misinterpreting it as carcinoma.

MICROSCOPIC FEATURES
■ Nephrogenic metaplasia occurs in the epithelium or the subepithelium, close to the urothelium (Figure 1-49). When involving the surface, a papillary appearance may form.
■ Acute and chronic inflammation is typically associated with nephrogenic metaplasia.
■ Lesions are composed of small tubules with a variety of histologic appearances. The tubules can be very small to dilated, have a flattened lining mimicking small vessels, be hobnailed, plump, or can have a signet ring appearance (Figure 1-50).

(text continued on page 46)

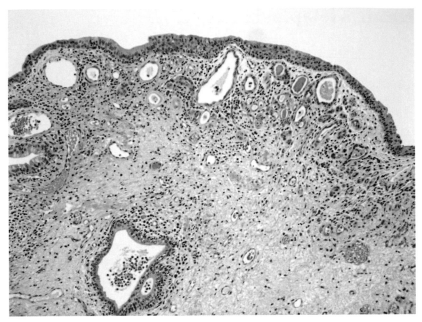

FIGURE 1-49

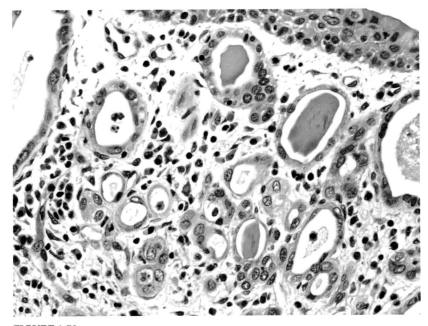

FIGURE 1-50

FIGURE 1-49   Within the prostatic urethra, nephrogenic metaplasia is seen directly beneath the urothelium.

FIGURE 1-50   Nephrogenic metaplasia is composed of small to dilated tubules with a plump, flattened, hobnailed, or signet ring lining.

Nephrogenic Metaplasia *(continued)*

- The tubules may be empty or can be filled with dense eosinophilic material, resembling thyroid. An eosinophilic rim of hyaline material may circumscribe the tubules.
- Nuclei may have visible nucleoli but lack macronucleoli. Mitotic figures are usually absent (Figure 1-51).

ANCILLARY STUDIES

- AMACR, CK7, PAX2, and PAX8 are positive in nephrogenic metaplasia while p63 and HMWK are variably expressed or are negative (Figure 1-52). Weak reactivity may be seen using PSA and PSAP. The partial expression overlap with prostatic adenocarcinoma is an important pitfall to recognize.

DIFFERENTIAL DIAGNOSIS

- Prostatic adenocarcinoma: Well-differentiated prostatic adenocarcinoma can be confused with nephrogenic metaplasia. Histologically, prostatic adenocarcinoma displays more prominent nucleomegaly and nucleoli than nephrogenic metaplasia, which frequently contains a variety of growth patterns unusual for carcinoma. Typical prostatic cancer can cause confusion as both lesions may have a similar expression pattern, with reactivity for AMACR but negative for p63. Use of PAX2 and/or PAX8 can be helpful as both will be positive in nephrogenic metaplasia and negative in prostatic adenocarcinoma. Additionally, CK7 will have diffuse expression in nephrogenic metaplasia and is usually weak to negative in most prostate cancers.

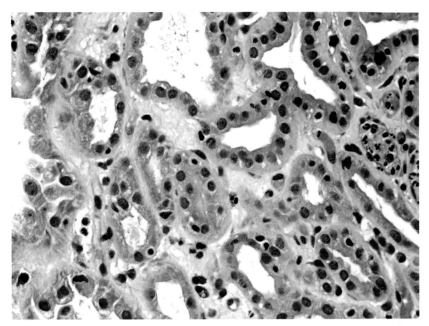

FIGURE 1-51

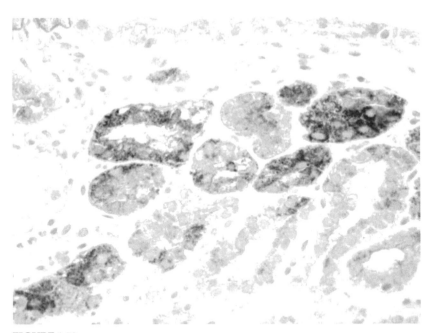

FIGURE 1-52

FIGURE 1-51   Here the nephrogenic metaplasia has a plump, eosinophilic lining that may be confused with prostatic adenocarcinoma. Nucleoli are seen, but these are pinpoint, not the macronucleoli seen in glands of prostate cancer.

FIGURE 1-52   AMACR is expressed in nephrogenic metaplasia, a key pitfall when differentiating this lesion from prostatic adenocarcinoma.

RADIATION CHANGE IN NONNEOPLASTIC GLANDS

DEFINITION
- Histologic alteration seen in nonneoplastic glands following radiation treatment.

CLINICAL FEATURES
- Patients with prostatic adenocarcinoma may receive radiation treatment via brachytherapy or external beam radiation.
- The histologic changes in the prostate can be seen for years after the radiation treatment.

MICROSCOPIC FEATURES
- Glands appear decreased in number, variable in size, and may appear infiltrative (Figure 1-53). Stroma can predominate the specimen.
- The majority of cells within a gland may be atypical basal cells.
- The glands can be a few layers thick or appear to have an increase in cell layers (Figure 1-54).

(text continued on page 50)

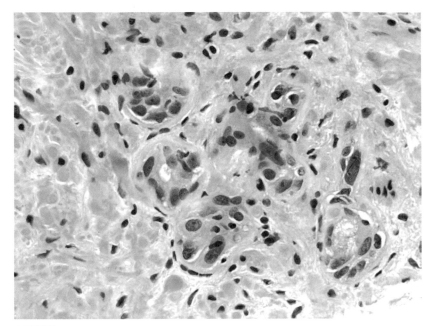

FIGURE 1-53

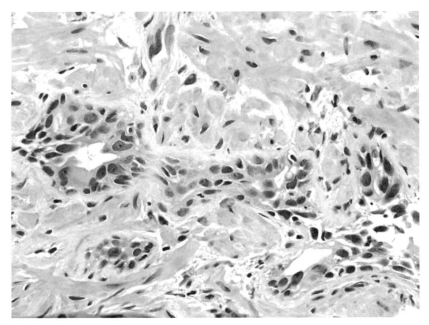

FIGURE 1-54

FIGURE 1-53 A cluster of postirradiated nonneoplastic glands has an infiltrative appearance with an increase in nuclear and nucleolar size. Basal cells are difficult to discriminate from apical cells. Unlike prostatic adenocarcinoma, nuclear overlap is present.

FIGURE 1-54 Nonneoplastic glands after radiation therapy show atrophy, with cellular stratification, nuclear pleomorphism, hyperchromasia, and prominent nucleoli.

Radiation Change in Nonneoplastic
Glands *(continued)*

■ Luminal borders may be straight and the glandular lumens can contain mucin (Figure 1-55). Atrophic glands, with a high nuclear-to-cytoplasm ratio, are typically present.

■ Squamous metaplasia, mucinous metaplasia, and Paneth cell-like change can be seen.

■ Nuclear atypia, pleomorphism, and hyperchromasia with variably prominent nucleoli are characteristic of radiation effect.

■ Radiation effect similar to other organs, including nuclear atypia of stromal cells, stromal fibrosis, and vascular hyalinization are usually identified.

ANCILLARY STUDIES

■ Basal cell markers, including p63 and HMWK, will highlight basal cells and AMACR will be weak to negative (Figure 1-56).

DIFFERENTIAL DIAGNOSIS

■ Prostatic adenocarcinoma: Residual adenocarcinoma with radiation change may be admixed with histologically altered nonneoplastic glands. Many histologic features, such as nucleomegaly, nucleolar prominence, intraluminal mucin, and straight luminal borders, are not reliable for diagnosing carcinoma in the postirradiation setting. Post radiation therapy, nonneoplastic glands may show more cellular stratification and denser cytoplasm than carcinoma. Immunostains are recommended for cases with an uncertain diagnosis, with p63, HMWK, and AMACR demonstrating the opposite staining pattern in these two entities.

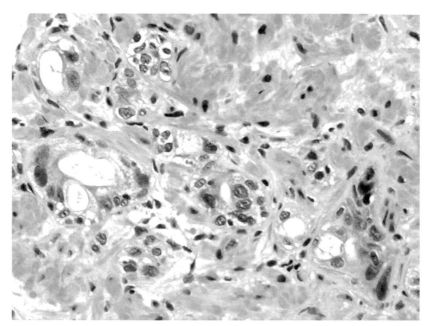

FIGURE 1-55

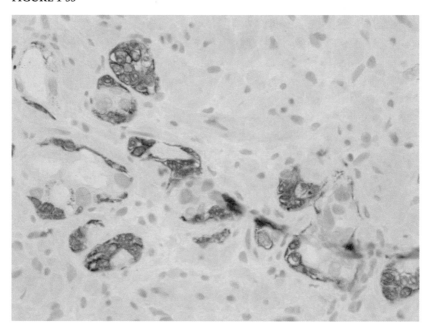

FIGURE 1-56

FIGURE 1-55 Small infiltrative-appearing postradiation glands with straight luminal borders, mucin, and prominent nucleoli mimic prostatic adenocarcinoma. Additionally, basal cells with supranuclear vacuolization are seen.

FIGURE 1-56 Immunostaining of the tissue in Figure 1-55 is shown. Basal cell markers, p63 (brown) and CK5 (brown), are positive while AMACR (pink) is weak to negative in these nonneoplastic glands status postradiation therapy.

NORMAL STRUCTURES WHICH MAY MIMIC ADENOCARCINOMA

Seminal Vesicles/Ejaculatory Ducts

DEFINITION
■ Seminal vesicles are paired, tubular accessory glands, which join the vas deferentia to form the ejaculatory ducts and enter the urethra at the verumontanum.

CLINICAL FEATURES
■ Secretes the majority of the ejaculatory fluid.
■ Secretions nourish sperm and modulate spermatic motility.
■ Main clinical relevance is to differentiate seminal vesicle/ejaculatory duct epithelium from prostatic adenocarcinoma within needle biopsy specimens.

MICROSCOPIC FEATURES
■ Dilated larger, central lumens surrounded by smaller glands. The smaller glands may have a crowded, infiltrative appearance (Figure 1-57).
■ Seminal vesicle ducts are surrounded by a well-formed muscular wall while the ejaculatory ducts are circumscribed by loose connective tissue.
■ Two types of cell layers are present. The inner layer is composed of cells with large nuclei, some of which can be quite pleomorphic, have prominent nucleoli, and are hyperchromatic.
■ Nuclear pseudoinclusions may be present (Figure 1-58).

(text continued on page 54)

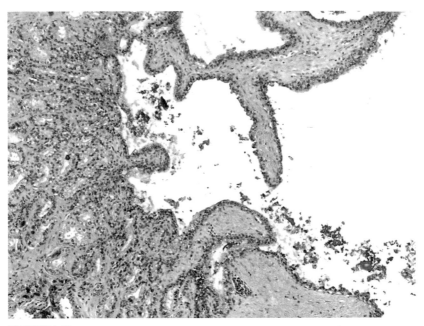

FIGURE 1-57

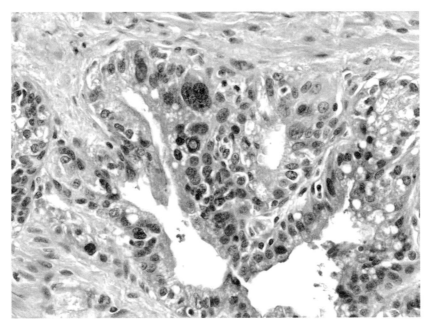

FIGURE 1-58

FIGURE 1-57   A dilated lumen is surrounded by crowded, smaller glands radiating from the large lumen.

FIGURE 1-58   Nucleomegaly, hyperchromasia and nuclear pseudoinclusions are present in seminal vesicle epithelium, unlike prostatic adenocarcinoma.

Chapter 1: Nonneoplastic Conditions   *53*

Seminal Vesicles/Ejaculatory Ducts *(continued)*

- Golden-brown lipofuscin cytoplasmic pigment can be seen (Figure 1-59).
- Often present at the end of a biopsy core.
- Mucosal and submucosal amyloid may be present (Figure 1-60).

ANCILLARY STUDIES
- Basal cell markers (p63 and HMWK) will highlight basal cells and AMACR will be weak to negative.
- PAX2 (paired box gene 2) and PAX8 (paired box gene 8) are positive.
- PSA and PSAP can show expression.
- ERG (Ets-related gene) is negative.

DIFFERENTIAL DIAGNOSIS
- Prostatic adenocarcinoma: Two types of cell layers are present in seminal vesicle/ejaculatory duct epithelium, which can be confirmed using basal cell markers while adenocarcinoma will only have one cell type. AMACR will be weak to negative in seminal vesicles, unlike carcinoma. Nuclear pleomorphism is greater in seminal vesicles than what is usually seen in prostatic adenocarcinoma.
- High-grade prostatic intraepithelial neoplasia: Nucleomegaly and nuclear pleomorphism are less in high-grade prostatic intraepithelial neoplasia than in seminal vesicle mucosa. Additionally, nuclear pseudoinclusions and cytoplasmic lipofuscin will not be present in high-grade prostatic intraepithelial neoplasia.

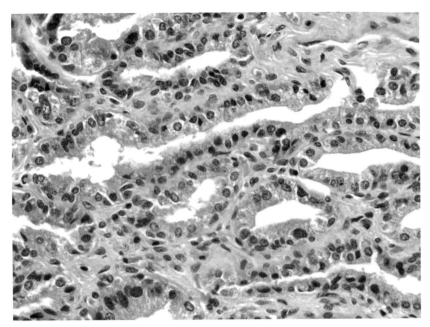

FIGURE 1-59

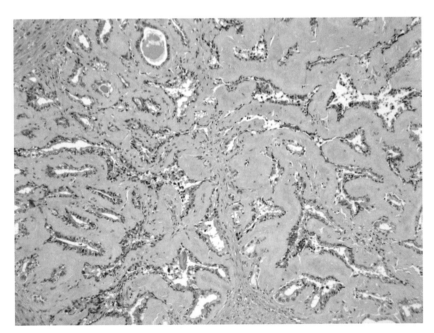

FIGURE 1-60

FIGURE 1-59   Course golden-brown lipofuscin is a histologic feature within seminal vesicle epithelium, which is helpful in the discrimination from prostatic adenocarcinoma.

FIGURE 1-60   Submucosal acellular light pink material, consistent with amyloid, is seen in this seminal vesicle.

Ganglia/Paraganglia/Peripheral Nerves

DEFINITION
- A ganglion is a mass of neuron cell bodies and glial cells.
- Paraganglia are clusters of extra-adrenal neuroendocrine chromaffin cells and sustentacular supporting cells.
- Peripheral nerves provide sympathetic and parasympathetic innervation.

CLINICAL FEATURES
- These are normal structures that are relevant only to differentiate them from prostatic adenocarcinoma.

MICROSCOPIC FEATURES
- A ganglion is composed of ganglion cells, which are large, have abundant pale eosinophilic cytoplasm, centrally located nuclei, very prominent nucleoli and may have granular, brownish Nissl substance at the periphery of the cell (Figure 1-61).
- A paraganglion is composed of nests of cells with clear to pale cytoplasm with small, dark, bland appearing nuclei. Flattened supportive sustentacular cells are usually inconspicuous (Figure 1-62).
- Peripheral nerve branches are composed of pale wavy cells with bland cytoplasm. Typically, larger cells that encircle or are within nerves represent prostatic adenocarcinoma. However, ganglion cells and nonneoplastic prostate glands may be found within and around nerves, mimicking prostatic adenocarcinoma (Figures 1-63 and 1-64).

ANCILLARY STUDIES
- Paraganglia are positive for synaptophysin and chromogranin and have S-100 reactivity in sustentacular cells.
- Ganglion cells and peripheral nerves are S-100 positive.
- Basal cell markers (p63 and HMWK), AMACR, and keratin are negative.

DIFFERENTIAL DIAGNOSIS
- Prostatic adenocarcinoma: In contrast to ganglion cells, prostatic adenocarcinoma has smaller, less uniform cells. Prostatic adenocarcinoma has larger nuclei and nucleoli compared to paraganglia. Immunostains can be performed if the diagnosis is uncertain.

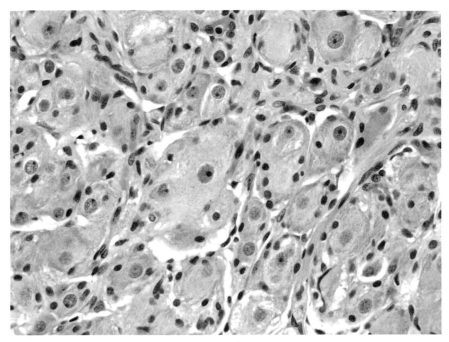

FIGURE 1-61

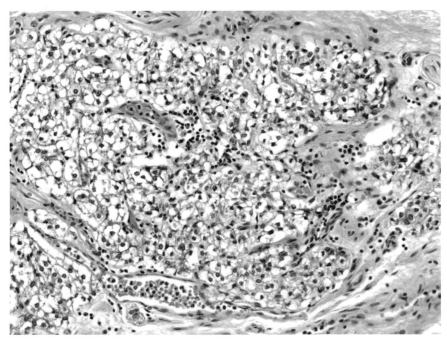

FIGURE 1-62

(continued)

FIGURE 1-61   A ganglion composed of cells that have very prominent nucleoli and abundant cytoplasm containing peripheral Nissl substance.

FIGURE 1-62   A paraganglion with cleared-out cells and hyperchromatic, bland nuclei.

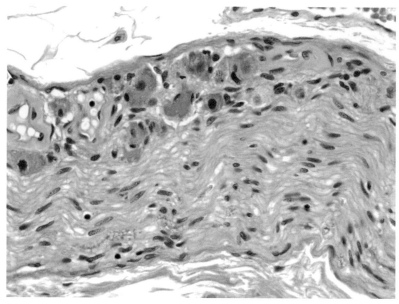

FIGURE 1-63

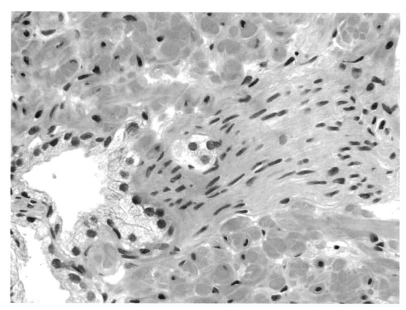

FIGURE 1-64

FIGURE 1-63 Ganglion cells cuffing a nerve can mimic prostatic adenocarcinoma.

FIGURE 1-64 A nonneoplastic gland touches and is entrapped within a nerve. This is a rare finding which can mimic carcinoma.

Cowper's Glands (Bulbourethral Glands)

DEFINITION
- Paired, pea-sized glands outside of the prostate, lateral to the apex.

CLINICAL FEATURES
- Produces lubricant secretions.
- Rarely seen in prostate biopsy specimens but may be encountered in transurethral resections or prostatectomy specimens.
- Must differentiate Cowper's glands from prostatic adenocarcinoma.

MICROSCOPIC FEATURES
- Typically located within skeletal muscle.
- Lobular configuration (Figure 1-65).
- Central spherical ducts lined by bland, cuboidal cells surrounded by small glands that are composed of mucin filled cells with basilar, compressed, hyperchromatic nuclei. The acini have small, inconspicuous lumina (Figure 1-66).

ANCILLARY STUDIES
- Periodic acid-Schiff with diastase (PAS-D) is positive in acini and negative in central ducts (Figure 1-67).
- Central ductal cells express HMWK while acini are predominately negative (Figure 1-68).
- PSA is negative and PSAP has variable reactivity.

DIFFERENTIAL DIAGNOSIS
- Prostatic adenocarcinoma: Foamy gland prostatic adenocarcinoma may mimic Cowper's glands but typically has larger, more open lumina with denser, slightly darker cytoplasm.
- Nonneoplastic conditions, including adenosis and mucinous metaplasia: Other nonneoplastic conditions may mimic Cowper's glands. For practical purposes, classification of these entities is not necessary. However, the extraprostatic location, particularly within skeletal muscle, will favor Cowper's glands, while an intraprostatic location will not.

(continued)

Cowper's Glands (Bulbourethral Glands) *(continued)*

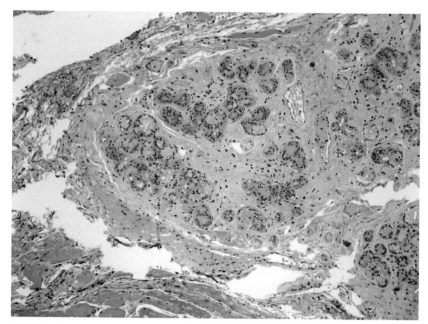

FIGURE 1-65

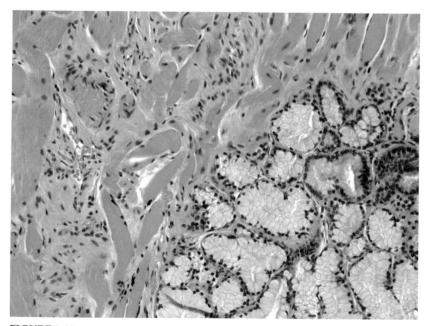

FIGURE 1-66

FIGURE 1-65 Cowper's glands within skeletal muscle in a prostatectomy specimen. A lobular configuration is seen.

FIGURE 1-66 Compact mucinous glands with small, to inconspicuous lumina are present, adjacent to skeletal muscle.

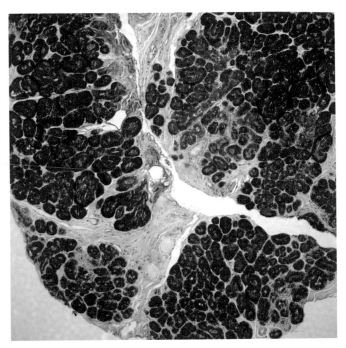

FIGURE 1-67

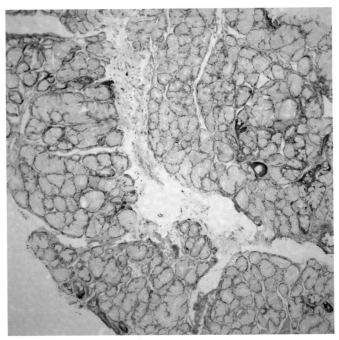

FIGURE 1-68

FIGURE 1-67   PAS-D is diffusely positive in the glands and is negative in a central duct.

FIGURE 1-68   HMWK is positive in central ducts and is variable in the acini, with many glands negative.

Colonic Glands

DEFINITION
■ Colonic glands are a normal finding in prostatic needle core biopsies.

CLINICAL FEATURES
■ The presence of colonic mucosa in needle core biopsies has no clinical relevance except to differentiate from prostatic adenocarcinoma.

MICROSCOPIC FEATURES
■ Typically, the colonic glands are present in a detached piece of tissue.
■ Rarely, the colonic mucosa is artifactually pushed into a prostatic needle core, usually only at one end of the core, or can be displaced into adipose tissue, mimicking extraprostatic extension (Figure 1-69).
■ Mucin is frequently seen, within goblet cells or extracellularly.
■ Nuclei are large and hyperchromatic (Figure 1-70).
■ Prominent nucleoli and mitotic figures are occasionally identified.

(*text continued on page 64*)

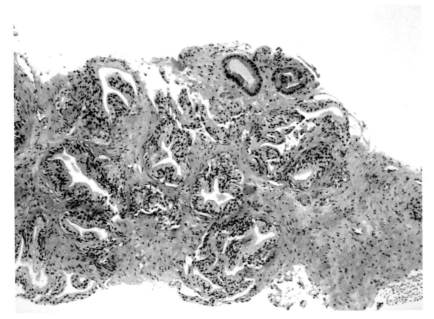

FIGURE 1-69

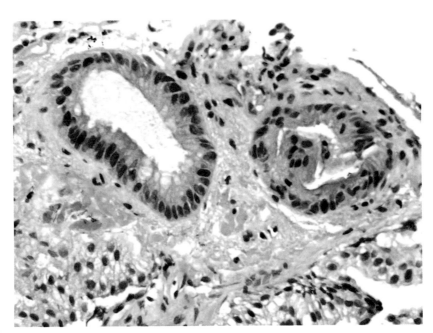

FIGURE 1-70

FIGURE 1-69   Two colonic glands pushed into the edge of this prostate needle core biopsy mimic prostatic adenocarcinoma.

FIGURE 1-70   The colonic glands from Figure 1-69 seen at higher magnification have hyperchromatic, enlarged nuclei similar to carcinoma.

Colonic Glands *(continued)*

ANCILLARY STUDIES
- PSA, PSAP, and basal cell markers (p63 and HMWK) are negative (Figure 1-71).
- CK20, CDX2 (caudal-type homeobox protein 2), and AMACR are positive (Figure 1-72).

DIFFERENTIAL DIAGNOSIS
- Prostatic adenocarcinoma: Prostatic adenocarcinoma will lack goblet cells. Colonic mucosa is typically detached. For rare difficult cases, immunohistochemical stains for colonic origin (CK20, CDX2) and prostatic origin (PSA, PSAP) are helpful.

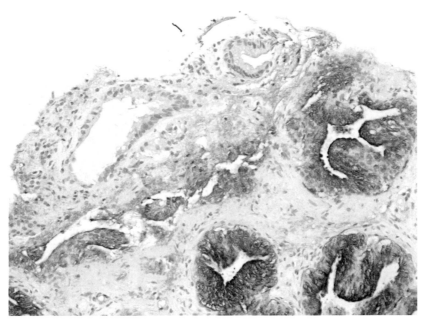

FIGURE 1-71

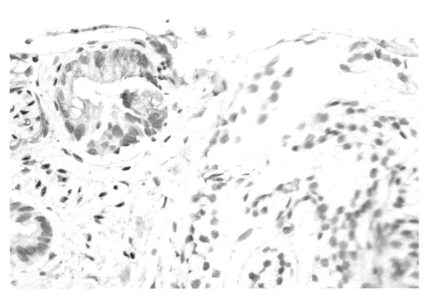

FIGURE 1-72

FIGURE 1-71   PSA is negative in the two colonic glands depicted in Figure 1-69 but is positive in the prostatic glands.

FIGURE 1-72   CK20 is positive in the colonic gland and is negative in the prostatic glands.

Premalignant Conditions and Prostate Carcinoma

2

High-Grade Prostatic Intraepithelial Neoplasia (HGPIN)

DEFINITION
- Premalignant condition with proliferation of epithelial cells with significant cytological and architectural atypia, including nuclear and nucleolar abnormalities.
- Confined to preexisting prostatic ducts and acini.
- Prostatic intraepithelial neoplasia (PIN) is graded from low grade to high grade.

CLINICAL FEATURES
- Low-grade PIN should not be diagnosed as the diagnosis of low-grade PIN is highly subjective and lacks clinical relevance.
- High-grade PIN (HGPIN) is more common in men with prostate cancer.
- Men with HGPIN on initial core biopsy have a higher risk of prostate carcinoma in the subsequent biopsy as compared to those without HGPIN.
- Risk of prostate cancer on first re-biopsy within 1 year following a diagnosis of HGPIN is related to the number of cores sampled.
- Men with low-grade PIN have no greater risk of finding prostate cancer with repeat biopsies.
- The predictive value for cancer of an initial diagnosis of HGPIN on needle biopsy has declined significantly (21%–36%), related to increased use of needle biopsy core sampling.

MICROSCOPIC FEATURES
- Low-grade PIN does not have prominent nucleoli while HGPIN has prominent nucleoli at 20× magnification.
- There are four architectural patterns of HGPIN: tufting, micropapillary, cribriform, and flat (Figure 2-1).
- HGPIN is more common in the peripheral zone of the prostate.
- HGPIN is often located adjacent to foci of cancer.
- Low power appearance of darker glands.
- Layer of crowded, pseudostratified secretory cells with cytological atypia, including nuclear irregularity, nucleomegaly, hyperchromasia, and prominent nucleoli at 20× (Figures 2-2 and 2-3).
- The chromatin pattern is coarse and clumpy.

(text continued on page 70)

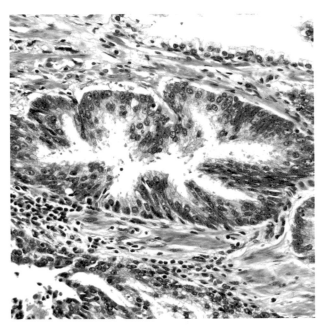

FIGURE 2-1

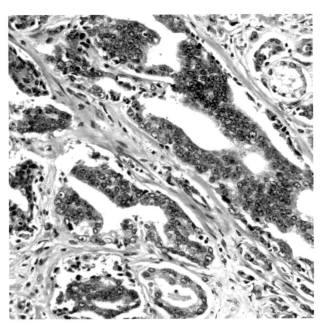

FIGURE 2-2

FIGURE 2-1 Morphological appearance of HGPIN with nuclear crowding and stratification. Note the darker cytoplasm as compared to adjacent benign glands.

FIGURE 2-2 HGPIN with nuclear crowding, stratification, and prominent nucleoli. Note the presence of atypical glands adjacent to focus of PIN. These may represent either out pouching of the HGPIN or a focus of microinvasive carcinoma.

Chapter 2: Premalignant Conditions and Prostate Carcinoma   *69*

High-Grade Prostatic Intraepithelial Neoplasia (HGPIN) (*continued*)

ANCILLARY STUDIES

■ Using the double-color triple-antibody (alpha-methylacyl-CoA racemase [AMACR], high molecular weight keratin [HMWK], and p63) cocktail, PIN will demonstrate patchy nuclear (p63) and cytoplasmic (HMWK) basal cell staining (brown) as well as cytoplasmic AMACR (pink) staining (Figure 2-4).

DIFFERENTIAL DIAGNOSIS

■ Normal prostatic anatomical structures such as central zone glands or seminal vesicle/ejaculatory ducts.
■ Benign lesions such as hyperplastic glands with reactive atypia or clear cell cribriform hyperplasia.
■ Prostate adenocarcinoma, cribriform pattern.
■ Intraductal carcinoma of the prostate.
■ Ductal adenocarcinoma.

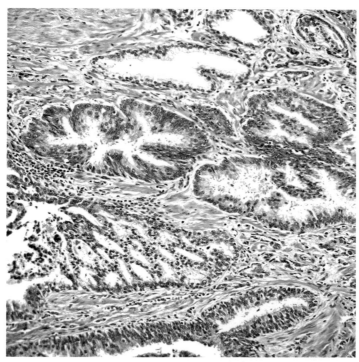

FIGURE 2-3

FIGURE 2-3   HGPIN with nuclear crowding, stratification, amphophilic cytoplasm, and prominent nucleoli. The epithelial cells proliferate giving the appearance of multilayering. Note the coarse pattern of the chromatin.

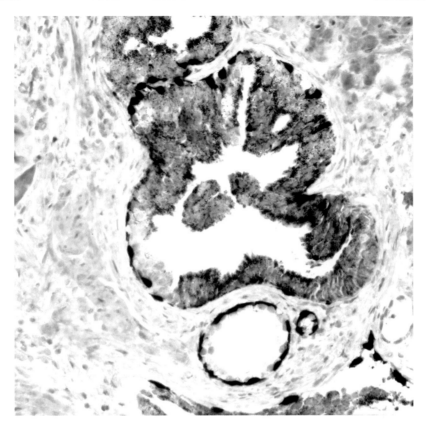

FIGURE 2-4

FIGURE 2-4   Using the double-color triple-antibody (AMACR, HMWK, and p63) cocktail, a focus of HGPIN demonstrates patchy nuclear (p63) and cytoplasmic (HMWK) basal cell staining (brown) as well as cytoplasmic AMACR staining (red).

Features of Prostatic Adenocarcinoma

DEFINITION
■ Acinar adenocarcinoma of the prostate is the most commonly diagnosed form of nonskin cancer in men in the United States.
■ The diagnosis of prostatic adenocarcinoma is based on a spectrum of luminal, architectural, nuclear, and cytoplasmic features.

CLINICAL FEATURES
■ Majority of the cancer cases in the United States are diagnosed in patients who are asymptomatic.
■ Age, race, and positive family history of prostate cancer are established risk factors.
■ Prostate cancer may be detected by abnormal digital rectal exam (DRE).
■ Elevation in serum prostate specific antigen (PSA) levels.
■ Treatment for prostate cancer depends on the overall Gleason grade of the disease and stage.
■ Treatments include active surveillance, surgery, radiation therapy, hormonal therapy, or cryotherapy.

MICROSCOPIC FEATURES
■ LUMINAL FEATURES
  ❑ Blue-tinged intraluminal wispy mucin (Figures 2-5 and 2-6).
  ❑ Crystalloids (Figure 2-7).
    • Usually rhomboid in shape with sharp edges (Figure 2-8).
    • Often seen in association with eosinophilic secretions.
    • May also be seen in foci of adenosis.
  ❑ Comedo-necrosis may be present in higher grade tumors.
  ❑ Lack of corpora amylacea.
  ❑ Eosinophilic secretions.
    • Usually granular (Figure 2-9).

(*text continued on page 76*)

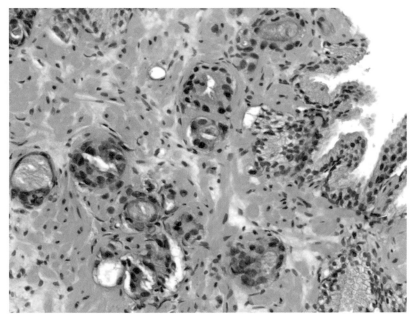

FIGURE 2-5

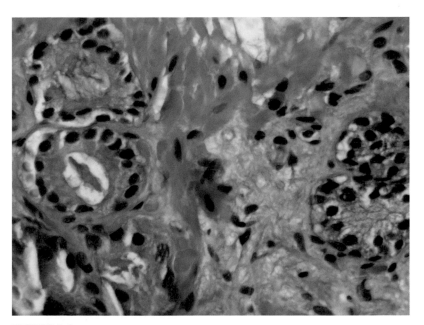

FIGURE 2-6

FIGURE 2-5   Presence of intraluminal blue mucin is a feature of prostatic adenocarcinoma, although some benign glands or benign mimickers of cancer may also possess intraluminal blue mucin.

FIGURE 2-6   Wispy intraluminal blue mucin in a malignant prostatic carcinoma gland with adjacent glands with some intraluminal pink secretions.

Chapter 2: Premalignant Conditions and Prostate Carcinoma   73

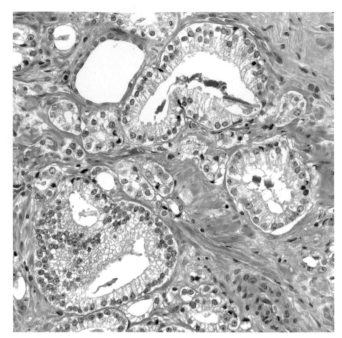

FIGURE 2-7

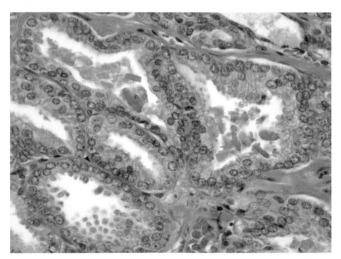

FIGURE 2-8

FIGURE 2-7   Prostatic adenocarcinoma glands with prominent intraluminal crystalloids.

FIGURE 2-8   Prostatic adenocarcinoma with prominent intraluminal crystalloids. Note the rhomboid shape of the crystals with sharp edges.

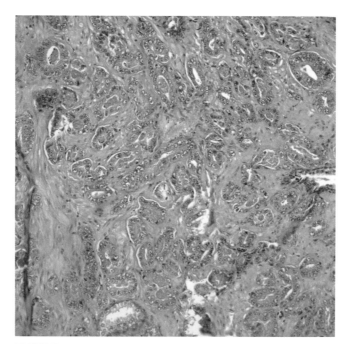

FIGURE 2-9

FIGURE 2-9 Prostate adenocarcinoma glands with granular intraluminal eosinophilic secretions.

Features of Prostatic Adenocarcinoma *(continued)*

■ ARCHITECTURAL FEATURES
   ❏ Well-differentiated tumors comprised of groups of well-formed glands (Figure 2-10).
   ❏ Poorly differentiated glands may appear as solid sheets of tumor or may have scattered single cells, or a prominent cribriform appearance (Figure 2-11).
   ❏ Malignant glands can be seen infiltrating amidst benign glands and can be seen on both sides of benign glands.
   ❏ Sharp luminal borders (Figure 2-12).
   ❏ Crowded collection of glands.

(text continued on page 78)

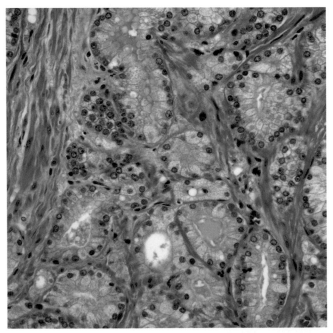

FIGURE 2-10

FIGURE 2-10   Well-differentiated prostatic adenocarcinoma with groups of well-formed glands.

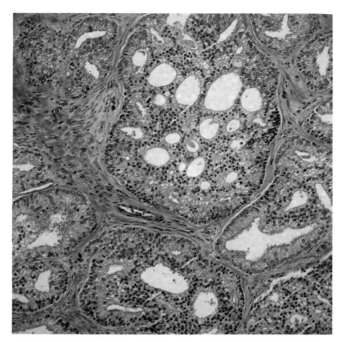

FIGURE 2-11

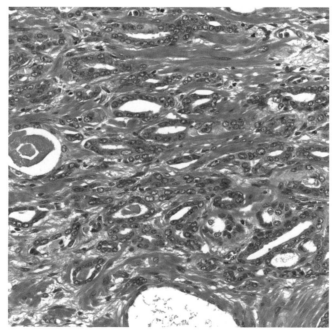

FIGURE 2-12

FIGURE 2-11   Prostatic adenocarcinoma with prominent cribriform appearance.

FIGURE 2-12   Prostatic adenocarcinoma with sharp luminal borders.

Chapter 2: Premalignant Conditions and Prostate Carcinoma   77

Features of Prostatic Adenocarcinoma *(continued)*

■ NUCLEAR FEATURES
- ❐ Enlarged nuclei (Figure 2-13).
- ❐ Hyperchromatic nuclei (Figure 2-13).
- ❐ Prominent nucleoli, often more than one (Figures 2-14 and 2-15).
- ❐ Often have chromatin clearing (Figure 2-15).
- ❐ May have mitosis.
- ❐ Lack of pleomorphic nuclei, except in rare cases.

(text continued on page 80)

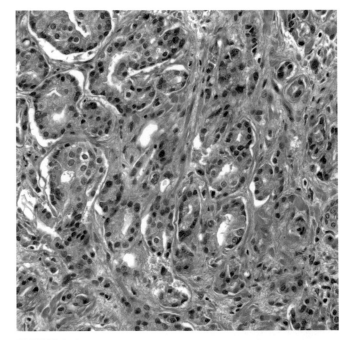

FIGURE 2-13

FIGURE 2-13 Prostatic adenocarcinoma with malignant glands with atypical nuclear features, including nucleomegaly and hyperchromatic nuclei.

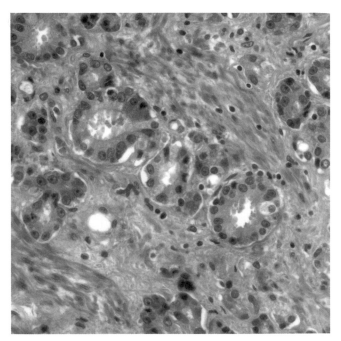

FIGURE 2-14

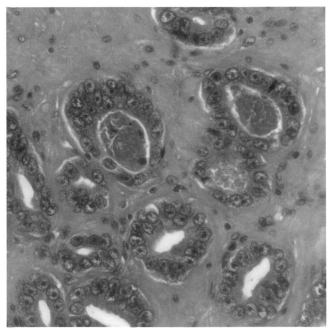

FIGURE 2-15

FIGURE 2-14   Prostatic adenocarcinoma with prominent nucleoli. The latter is a characteristic feature
of prostate carcinoma.

FIGURE 2-15   Prostatic adenocarcinoma with characteristic nuclear features, including prominent
nucleoli, some with more than one nucleolus, and chromatin clearing.

Chapter 2: Premalignant Conditions and Prostate Carcinoma

Features of Prostatic Adenocarcinoma (*continued*)

- Cytoplasmic features
  - ❑ Cells are cuboidal or columnar in shape, some with foamy appearance.
  - ❑ Amphophilic (darker) cytoplasm as compared to coexisting benign glands (Figure 2-16).
  - ❑ Lack of lipofuscin.
  - ❑ Lower grade carcinoma has paler cytoplasm.

PATHOGNOMONIC FEATURES OF PROSTATE CANCER
- Mucinous fibroplasia (collagenous micronodules).
  - ❑ Mucinous fibroplasia is a characteristic finding that may be seen in prostatic adenocarcinoma. It represents hyalinized eosinophilic material often intermingled with wispy blue mucin (Figures 2-17 and 2-18).

(*text continued on page 82*)

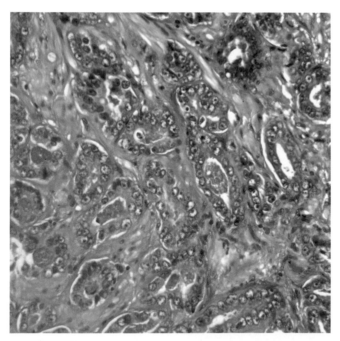

FIGURE 2-16

FIGURE 2-16   Prostate carcinoma glands with infiltrative appearance with prominent amphophilic cytoplasm and straight luminal borders.

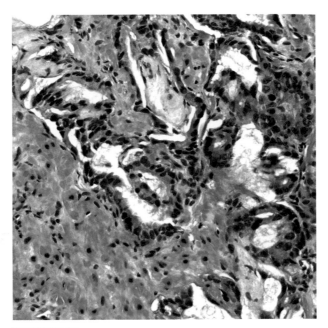

FIGURE 2-17

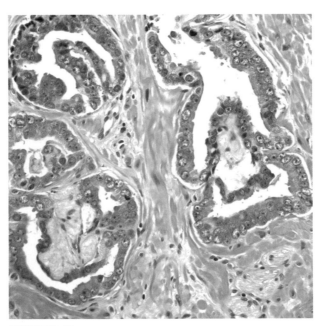

FIGURE 2-18

FIGURE 2-17   Characteristic presence of mucinous fibroplasia (collagen micronodules) in a case of infiltrating adenocarcinoma. A glomeruloid structure is formed by an intraluminal proliferation of malignant cells.

FIGURE 2-18   Mucinous fibroplasia (collagenous nodules), a pathognomonic feature of prostate cancer. This is often associated with blue mucin. Note the presence of crescent-shaped space resembling a renal glomerulus.

Features of Prostatic Adenocarcinoma *(continued)*

- Glomerulations
  - ☐ Glomerulations are another pathognomonic feature of prostate cancer. Essentially, this is a cribriform cellular luminal proliferation adherent to one of the poles.
  - ☐ The cribriform proliferation is surrounded by a crescentic space, closely resembling a renal glomerulus (Figures 2-19 and 2-20).
  - ☐ This finding is almost always diagnostic of carcinoma (Figures 2-19 and 2-20).
- Perineural invasion
  - ☐ Perineural invasion with carcinoma glands surrounding a nerve is a pathognomonic feature of prostate cancer (Figure 2-21).
  - ☐ Occasionally benign glands are seen abutting a nerve but they do not have circumferential extension entirely around a nerve (Figures 2-21–2-23).
  - ☐ Occasionally ganglion cells are present in close proximity to the nerve and may appear as cancer infiltrating a nerve bundle.

(text continued on page 85)

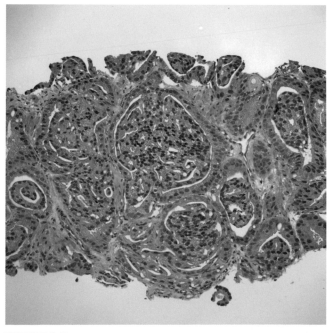

FIGURE 2-19

FIGURE 2-19   A glomeruloid formation is a pathognomonic finding in prostate cancer as seen on this prostate needle biopsy.

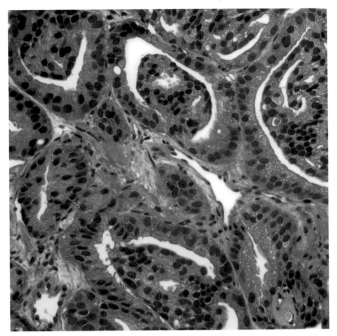

FIGURE 2-20

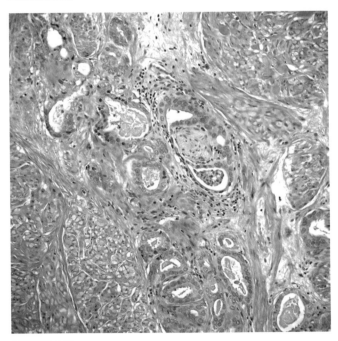

FIGURE 2-21

FIGURE 2-20   Glomerulation, a pathognomonic feature of prostate cancer, resembling a glomerulus from a kidney as seen in this case of prostate adenocarcinoma diagnosed on a needle biopsy.

FIGURE 2-21   Perineural invasion (circumferential involvement) is diagnostic of prostatic adenocarcinoma as seen here.

Features of Prostatic Adenocarcinoma (*continued*)

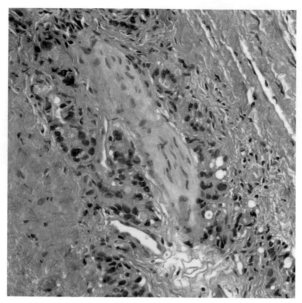

FIGURE 2-22

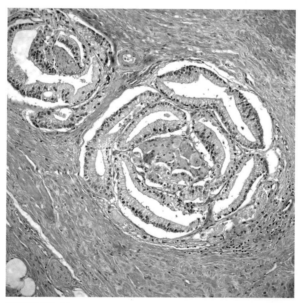

FIGURE 2-23

FIGURE 2-22   Prostate adenocarcinoma glands are seen tracking along a nerve with definite invasion of the nerve.

FIGURE 2-23   Perineural invasion is clearly seen in two clusters of malignant glands with circumferential involvement. Note the presence of ganglion cells and nerves intimately involved with the malignant cells.

ANCILLARY STUDIES
■ Absence of basal cell markers (p63, HMWK).
■ Positive AMACR expression (Figure 2-24).

DIFFERENTIAL DIAGNOSIS
■ Benign mimickers of prostate cancer, including benign prostatic anatomical structures such as seminal vesicles, Cowper glands, Verumontanum mucosal gland hyperplasia, and paraganglia.
■ Adenosis.
■ Mesonephric remnants.
■ Benign prostatic hyperplasia.
■ Atrophic glands, including ones with partial atrophy or complete atrophy.
■ Inflammation and reactive atypia.
■ Radiation atypia.
■ Proliferative lesions such as high-grade prostatic intraepithelial neoplasia.
■ Secondary high-grade tumors.

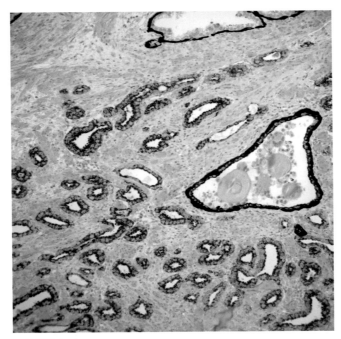

FIGURE 2-24

FIGURE 2-24   Use of ancillary testing such as the use of immunohistochemistry to evaluate basal cell markers (HMWK, p63) as well as AMACR (p504S). Cancer cells lack basal cells as seen here and are positive for AMACR.

Atypical Small Acinar Proliferation

DEFINITION
- Atypical small acinar proliferation (ASAP) is a descriptive term that should be restricted to lesions that are probably carcinoma but either lack definitive diagnostic features or are too small to be certain that they do not represent the edge of a benign lesion.
- ASAPs are either incompletely sampled cancer or benign glands with reactive atypia or atrophy.

CLINICAL FEATURES
- Found in approximately 2% to 5% of prostate needle biopsy specimens.
- A prostate biopsy is typically done following an abnormal digital rectal exam or an elevated serum PSA.
- Most frequently located in the peripheral zones of the prostate.
- Patients diagnosed with ASAP have a reported range of 17% to 60% probability of finding prostatic adenocarcinoma on a repeat biopsy.

MICROSCOPIC FEATURES
- Microscopic findings are similar to those of adenocarcinoma, with absence of basal cells in the atypical glands (Figure 2-25).
- Some helpful features are amphophilic cytoplasm, nucleomegaly, prominent nucleoli, intraluminal crystalloids, straight luminal borders, blue mucin, or pink secretions.
- Rarely mitotic figures may be seen (Figure 2-26).
- There are some findings that are suspicious for but not diagnostic for carcinoma. However, the suspicious focus of ASAP reveals a limitation that is either qualitative (degree of atypia) or quantitative (too few atypical glands), precluding a conclusive diagnosis of cancer (Figures 2-27 and 2-28).
- When the following histological findings are seen, a diagnosis of carcinoma should be made with caution:
  - ☐ Partial atrophy.
  - ☐ Acute inflammation.
  - ☐ Pale cytoplasm and atrophic features.
  - ☐ Crowded glands with lack of significant cytological atypia.
  - ☐ Lobular architecture.

ANCILLARY STUDIES
- Immunohistochemistry can be helpful in clarifying the diagnosis of ASAP on needle biopsies.
- HMWK (34βE12) (cytoplasmic) or p63 (nuclear) stains highlight the basal cell layer of prostatic acini (Figure 2-29).
- AMACR (P504S) serves as a positive immunostain to aid in the diagnosis of cancer (Figures 2-29 and 2-30).

DIFFERENTIAL DIAGNOSIS
- Prostate adenocarcinoma——The glands should have sufficient quantitative and qualitative features of malignancy.
- Benign mimickers of cancer such as partial atrophy, complete atrophy, inflammation, metaplasia, hyperplasia, or adenosis.
- Atypical glands adjacent to a focus of high-grade prostatic intraepithelial neoplasia.
- Benign anatomical structures such as seminal vesicles, paraganglia, or colonic mucosa.

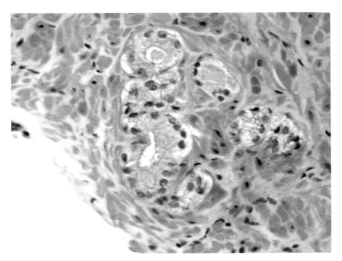

FIGURE 2-25

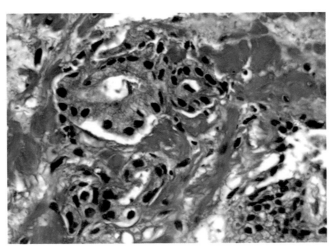

FIGURE 2-26

FIGURE 2-25 ASAP-Small focus of atypical glands with pale cytoplasm, moderate cytological atypia and somewhat prominent nucleoli. Overall, these findings are suspicious but not diagnostic for carcinoma.

FIGURE 2-26 ASAP suspicious for, but not diagnostic of, cancer. The cytoplasm is amphophilic. Overall, this lesion lacks sufficient cytological atypia to warrant a diagnosis of carcinoma.

Atypical Small Acinar Proliferation (*continued*)

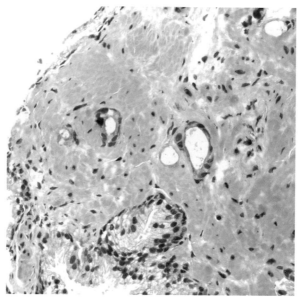

FIGURE 2-27

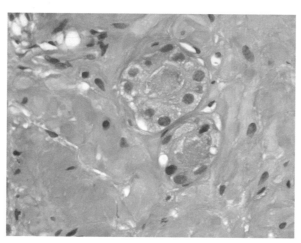

FIGURE 2-28

FIGURE 2-27   ASAP suspicious for, but not diagnostic of cancer. There are a handful of glands with significant atrophy. It is difficult to assess for nuclear atypia and there is a lack of prominent nucleoli. This may represent a small focus of atrophic prostatic adenocarcinoma, but, overall, this lesion lacks sufficient qualitative atypia to warrant a diagnosis of carcinoma.

FIGURE 2-28   ASAP. This lesion is not diagnostic of cancer because it has the appearance of a focus of partial atrophy. Also, the cytoplasm is pale and the number of glands is too few. Overall, this lesion lacks sufficient cytological atypia to warrant a diagnosis of carcinoma. Even if this lesion is negative for basal cell markers (p63, HMWK), it would be difficult to diagnose this as carcinoma.

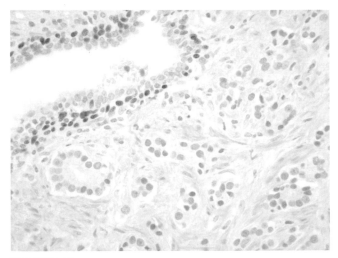

FIGURE 2-29

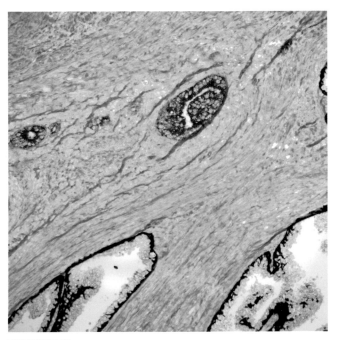

FIGURE 2-30

FIGURE 2-29 Occasionally, immunostains may be helpful in assessing foci of atypical glands which otherwise lack sufficient features of cancer. A needle biopsy shows a focus of small-caliber atypical glands with an infiltrative appearance, which, on immunohistochemistry with the basal cell marker p63, reveals absence of basal cells, thereby confirming a diagnosis of prostatic adenocarcinoma Gleason 3 + 3 = 6.

FIGURE 2-30 ASAP suspicious for, but not diagnostic of, cancer. Even though these three to four glands are negative for basal cell markers (p63, HMWK) and are positive for AMACR, the number of glands is too few, and, overall, there is a lack of sufficient cytological atypia to warrant a diagnosis of carcinoma.

Chapter 2: Premalignant Conditions and Prostate Carcinoma   *89*

Acinar Adenocarcinoma, Gleason Grading

DEFINITION
- Gleason grading is the most commonly used system for classifying the histologic characteristics of prostate cancer, utilizing the glandular architecture of the tumor for assessing tumor grade. This type of grading scheme in which an emphasis is placed on architectural patterns makes Gleason grading system fairly novel among other types of grading systems in pathology.

CLINICAL FEATURES
- Proposed by Donald F. Gleason in 1966.
- Recommended by World Health Organization in 1993.
- The system was updated at a 2005 consensus conference of international experts in urological pathology.
- Correlates well with prognosis.
- Rather than assigning the worst grade as the grade of the carcinoma, the grade was defined as the sum of the two most common grade patterns and reported as the Gleason score.
- Prostatic adenocarcinoma with a high Gleason score (8–10) is the most aggressive form of prostate cancer.

MICROSCOPIC FEATURES
- Based on glandular architecture.
- Nuclear atypia is not evaluated.
- The grading system is based on an assessment of the most common pattern and the second-most common pattern and assigning a grade between 1 and 5 to each pattern.
- Gleason grade is defined as the sum of the two most common grade patterns and reported as the Gleason score (e.g., 3 + 3 = 6) (Figure 2-31).
- A Gleason grade is based on the degree of differentiation of the tumor.
- A Gleason grade of 1 is most well-differentiated while a Gleason grade of 5 represents most poorly differentiated.
- Gleason scores range as follows:
  - ❑ Gleason score of 2 to 4: Well differentiated.
  - ❑ Gleason score of 5 to 7: Moderately differentiated.
  - ❑ Gleason score of 8 to 10: Poorly differentiated.
- Gleason grade 1—Nodules of closely-packed, uniform well-formed glands; inconspicuous nucleoli.
- Gleason grade 2—Nodule of glands, loosely-packed, minimal infiltration.
- Gleason grade 3—Most common pattern; infiltrating appearance; tumor infiltrates between benign glands (Figures 2-32, 2-33, and 2-34).
- Gleason grade 4—Poorly-formed or fused glands or clear cytoplasm with a dot-like nucleus (hypernephroid pattern); cribriform architecture (Figures 2-35, 2-36, 2-37, and 2-38).

(*text continued on page 96*)

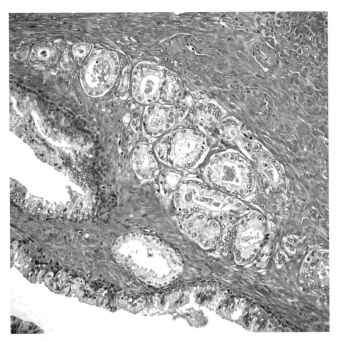

FIGURE 2-31

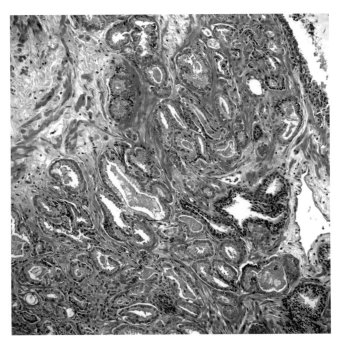

FIGURE 2-32

FIGURE 2-31   Prostatic adenocarcinoma, Gleason score 3 + 3 = 6 with an infiltrative growth pattern, with small to medium-sized malignant glands adjacent to benign glands.

FIGURE 2-32   Prostate needle biopsy showing prostatic adenocarcinoma, Gleason score 3 + 4 = 7. The Gleason pattern 4 glands are fused and poorly formed.

Chapter 2: Premalignant Conditions and Prostate Carcinoma   *91*

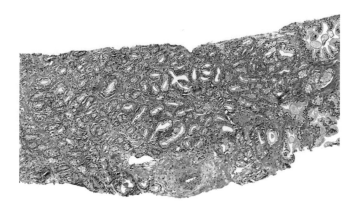

FIGURE 2-33

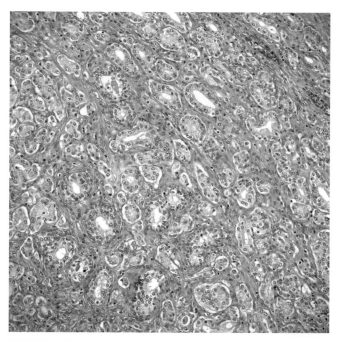

FIGURE 2-34

FIGURE 2-33   Low power view of a prostate needle biopsy with prostatic adenocarcinoma, Gleason score 3 + 4 = 7 with fused malignant glands (Gleason pattern 4) admixed with well formed, infiltrating glands (Gleason pattern 3). The dominant component is Gleason pattern 3 and hence this is graded as Gleason score of 3 + 4 = 7.

FIGURE 2-34   A section from a radical prostatectomy specimen showing a field comprising of prostatic adenocarcinoma, Gleason score 3 + 3 = 6 with well-formed, small-to-medium-sized infiltrating glands.

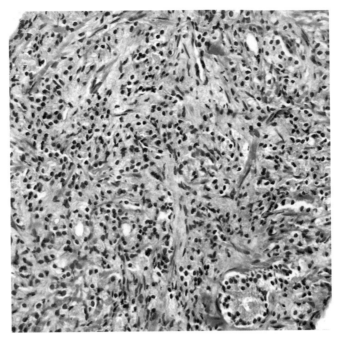

FIGURE 2-35

FIGURE 2-35   High power view of a field representing prostatic adenocarcinoma with a Gleason score of 4 + 5 = 9 diagnosed on a needle biopsy. There are Gleason patterns 3, 4, and 5 present, including focal area with solid sheet of neoplastic cells with no indication of lumen formation. Because this is a biopsy with Gleason patterns 3, 4, and 5, this should be graded overall as high grade with a primary Gleason pattern 4 and a secondary (highest grade) Gleason pattern of 5.

(continued)

Chapter 2: Premalignant Conditions and Prostate Carcinoma   93

Acinar Adenocarcinoma, Gleason Grading (continued)

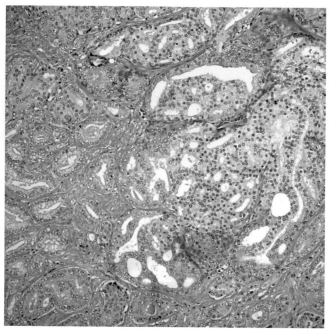

FIGURE 2-36

FIGURE 2-36 Prostatic adenocarcinoma diagnosed on a needle biopsy, Gleason score 4 + 3 = 7. The primary Gleason pattern is 4 with fused malignant glands, predominantly cribriform pattern and with a secondary Gleason pattern of 3 represented by infiltrating well-formed malignant glands of small to medium size.

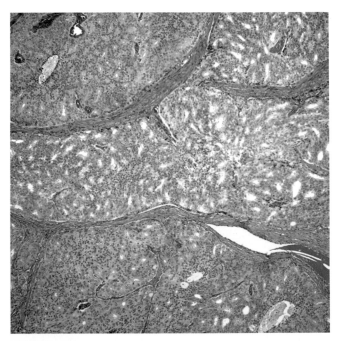

FIGURE 2-37

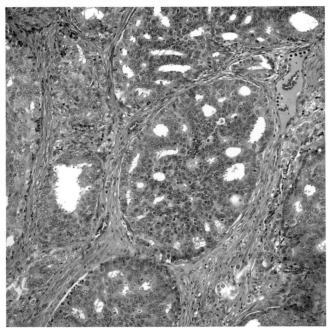

FIGURE 2-38

FIGURE 2-37 Prostatic adenocarcinoma diagnosed on a section from a radical prostatectomy specimen, Gleason score 4 + 4 = 8. The primary and secondary Gleason patterns are 4 with fused malignant glands, predominantly cribriform pattern.

FIGURE 2-38 Prostatic adenocarcinoma, Gleason score 4 + 4 = 8 diagnosed on a needle biopsy with cribriform neoplastic glands.

(*continued*)

Chapter 2: Premalignant Conditions and Prostate Carcinoma   *95*

Acinar Adenocarcinoma, Gleason Grading (*continued*)

- Gleason grade 5—Sheets or cords of cells with no or minimal gland formation; single infiltrative cells; signet-ring cells; cribriform architecture; comedonecrosis (Figures 2-39, 2-40, 2-41, and 2-42).
- Tertiary Gleason grade.
- Gleason grading of variants of prostate carcinoma.
- Gleason grading of prostate carcinoma which has been treated with hormone or radiation therapy.
- Based on the modified Gleason scoring system proposed in 2005:
  - ❏ Gleason score 2 to 4 should rarely be diagnosed on needle biopsy.
  - ❏ Certain patterns originally considered to be Gleason pattern 3 are now considered Gleason pattern 4.
  - ❏ All cribriform carcinomas should be graded pattern 4.

(*text continued on page 98*)

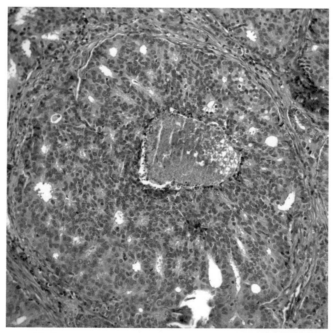

FIGURE 2-39

FIGURE 2-39   Prostatic adenocarcinoma, Gleason pattern 5 with cribriform gland and central necrosis (comedonecrosis).

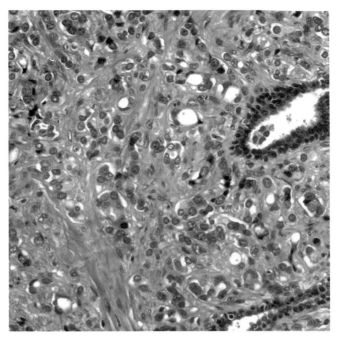

FIGURE 2-40

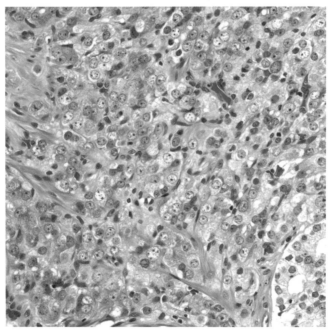

FIGURE 2-41

FIGURE 2-40   Prostatic adenocarcinoma, Gleason score 4 + 5 = 9 with single cells (Gleason pattern 5) admixed with poorly formed glands (Gleason pattern 4) some with no indication of lumen formation.

FIGURE 2-41   Prostatic adenocarcinoma, with an overall Gleason score of 5 + 4 = 9, predominantly comprising of single cells with a few poorly formed glands representing Gleason pattern 4.

Acinar Adenocarcinoma, Gleason Grading (continued)

ANCILLARY STUDIES

■ Immunohistochemistry may be helpful in separating carcinoma from benign mimickers of cancer.

■ Prostate cancer lacks basal cells (p63, HMWK) and stains strongly with AMACR.

DIFFERENTIAL DIAGNOSIS

■ Benign mimickers of cancer such as adenosis, partial atrophy, complete atrophy, hyperplasia, or normal anatomical structures such as Cowper's glands or seminal vesicles.

■ Granulomatous inflammation may mimic high Gleason grade cancer such as pattern 5.

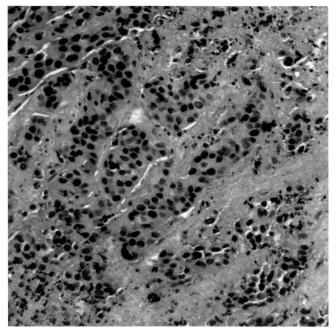

FIGURE 2-42

FIGURE 2-42   Prostatic adenocarcinoma, Gleason score 5 + 5 = 10 with solid sheet of neoplastic cells, some of which are single. There is no indication of lumen formation.

Acinar Adenocarcinoma, Treatment Effect

DEFINITION
- Both benign prostate and prostatic adenocarcinoma have a spectrum of morphological changes which occur after treatment with hormone or radiation therapy. A Gleason grade is not assigned to prostatic carcinoma with therapy-related changes.

CLINICAL FEATURES
- Radiation-induced changes.
  - The changes to prostatic tissue caused by radiation are highly variable and depend on the method used (brachytherapy vs. external beam), dose and duration of the radiation.
  - Following treatment, it is important for the urologist to indicate history of androgen deprivation or radiation therapy to enable the pathologist to carefully evaluate for the changes induced by treatment.
  - Radiation treatment is a treatment selected by 20% to 25% of men with prostate cancer.
  - Radiation treatment may be provided by brachytherapy or external beam radiation.
  - The changes to prostatic tissue caused by radiation are highly variable and depend on the method used (brachytherapy vs. external beam), dose and duration of the radiation.
- Hormone-induced changes.
  - Hormonal therapy (also known as endocrine or androgen-deprivation therapy) is usually the treatment of choice for disseminated prostate cancer.
  - Androgen deprivation may be done by orchiectomy, antiandrogens, 5 alpha-reductase or gonadotropin-releasing hormone antagonists.
  - Hormone therapy is used to shrink tumor size before surgery or to treat hyperplasia.
  - Hormonal therapy is also used in locally advanced disease.

(text continued on page 100)

Acinar Adenocarcinoma, Treatment Effect (continued)

MICROSCOPIC FEATURES
RADIATION THERAPY

■ Radiation effect on benign glands.

❏ Benign prostate with radiation therapy effect shows acinar atrophy with distortion and decrease in the number of glands (Figure 2-43).

❏ The secretory glands shrink in size and may have a flat appearance.

❏ Glands are smaller with occasional pyknotic nuclei while several nuclei appear enlarged and hyperchromatic with smudgy chromatin (Figures 2-44 and 2-45).

❏ May have urothelial metaplasia, basal cell hyperplasia, and squamous metaplasia.

❏ Stroma may contain scattered chronic inflammation infiltrates.

(*text continued on page 102*)

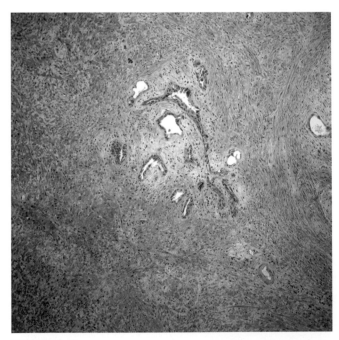

FIGURE 2-43

FIGURE 2-43　Benign prostatic tissue with pronounced radiation therapy effect showing prominent acinar atrophy with distortion and decrease in the number of glands. The glands continue to maintain their lobular architecture.

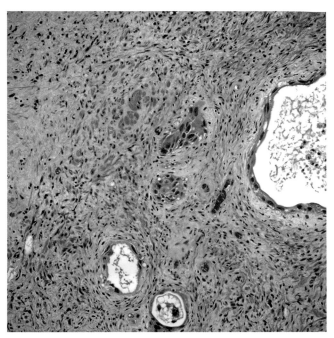

FIGURE 2-44

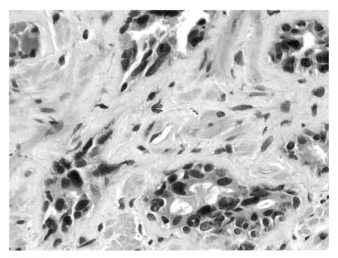

FIGURE 2-45

FIGURE 2-44   Benign prostate with radiation therapy effect. Note the atrophic and shrunken glands with prominent squamous metaplasia and an adjacent dilated gland with substantial atrophic changes.

FIGURE 2-45   Benign prostatic tissue from a patient with obstructive urinary symptoms and a past history of prostatic adenocarcinoma which has been treated with radiation therapy. Note that several nuclei appear enlarged and hyperchromatic with smudgy chromatin.

Acinar Adenocarcinoma, Treatment Effect (*continued*)

- ■ Radiation effect on malignant glands.
  - ❐ Prostatic adenocarcinoma with radiation therapy effect is highly variable and includes smaller glands which are poorly formed glands and may have single cells.
  - ❐ Cytoplasm is with vacuoles and nuclei are pyknotic (Figures 2-46 and 2-47).
  - ❐ The glands decrease number but may continue to have an infiltrative appearance and lack basal cell layers (Figure 2-48).
  - ❐ The malignant glands may retain some of the features of prostatic adenocarcinoma, including the presence of blue mucin and pink secretions.
  - ❐ A Gleason grade is not assigned to cancer which shows treatment effect.
  - ❐ Neoplastic glands lack basal cells and are positive for AMACR (Figure 2-49).

(*text continued on page 104*)

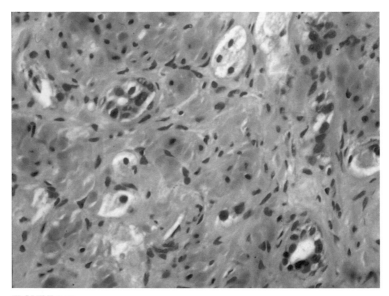

FIGURE 2-46

FIGURE 2-46   Prostatic adenocarcinoma with radiation therapy effect. The glands have an infiltrative appearance. Note the neoplastic cells have prominent vacuolated cytoplasm with pyknotic nuclei.

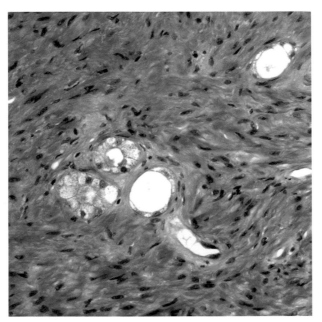

FIGURE 2-47

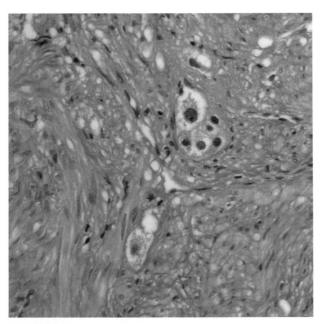

FIGURE 2-48

FIGURE 2-47   Prostatic adenocarcinoma with radiation therapy with poorly formed glands with vacuolated cytoplasm and pyknotic nuclei. Note the prominent stromal fibrosis. There is no nuclear pleomorphism.

FIGURE 2-48   Prostatic tissue from a patient who underwent transurethral resection of prostate to alleviate the symptoms of benign prostatic hyperplasia. This section shows scattered atypical glands with some features of prostatic adenocarcinoma with radiation treatment effect. Note the prominent vacuolation and the poorly formed glands.

Chapter 2: Premalignant Conditions and Prostate Carcinoma   *103*

Acinar Adenocarcinoma, Treatment Effect *(continued)*

HORMONAL THERAPY

■ Hormonal effect on benign glands.

❑ Benign prostate with hormonal therapy effect tends to have more stroma and fewer glands.

❑ Glands appear smaller, ovoid or round and atrophic with small pyknotic nuclei, inconspicuous nucleoli, and cytoplasmic clearing.

❑ May have basal cell hyperplasia, epithelial cell vacuolation, and squamous metaplasia (Figure 2-50).

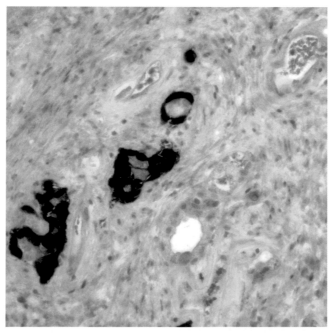

FIGURE 2-49

FIGURE 2-49   Prostate carcinoma with radiation changes, including poorly formed glands. An immunostain for basal cell markers (p63, HMWK) may be useful in further characterization of this lesion as prostatic adenocarcinoma with therapy-related changes. Note the weak AMACR expression in the malignant glands.

■ Hormonal effect on malignant glands.
  ❒ Prostatic adenocarcinoma with hormonal therapy effect tends to have shrunken atrophic glands or, more commonly, widely dispersed single cells resembling histiocytes (Figures 2-51 and 2-52).
  ❒ Malignant glands have pyknotic nuclei, inconspicuous nucleoli, clear cytoplasm, and foamy or vacuolated cytoplasm (Figures 2-52 and 2-53).
  ❒ Stroma may be edematous or inflamed.
  ❒ May see ruptured malignant glands with mucin extravasation.
  ❒ A Gleason grade is not assigned to cancer which shows treatment effect.

(text continued on page 108)

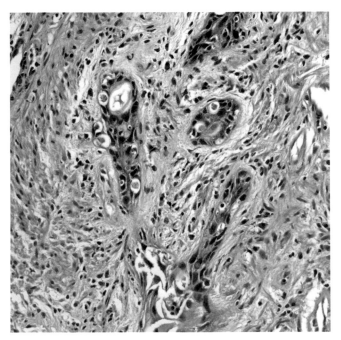

FIGURE 2-50

FIGURE 2-50   Benign prostate with hormone therapy effect. Note the prominent squamous metaplasia with reactive atypia and prominent epithelial cell vacuolation. No malignant glands are apparent in this field of view.

Chapter 2: Premalignant Conditions and Prostate Carcinoma   *105*

Acinar Adenocarcinoma, Treatment Effect (*continued*)

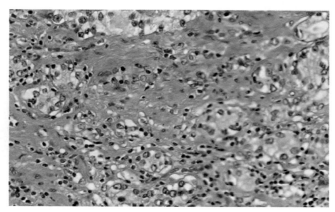

FIGURE 2-51

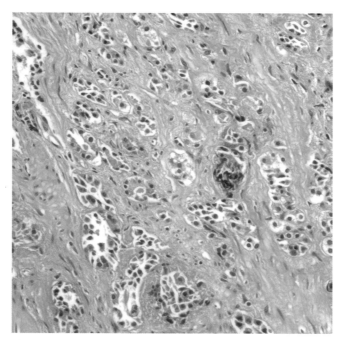

FIGURE 2-52

FIGURE 2-51   Prostate adenocarcinoma with hormone therapy-related changes. Note the presence of single cells with an appearance resembling that of histiocytes.

FIGURE 2-52   Prostate adenocarcinoma with hormone therapy-related changes. Malignant glands have pyknotic nuclei, inconspicuous nucleoli, clear cytoplasm, and foamy or vacuolated cytoplasm.

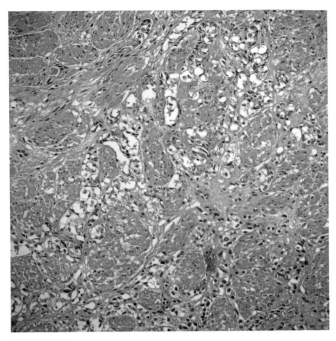

FIGURE 2-53

FIGURE 2-53   Prostate adenocarcinoma with hormone therapy-related changes, including widely
scattered single cells and atrophic-appearing glands.

Acinar Adenocarcinoma, Treatment Effect *(continued)*

ANCILLARY STUDIES

■ Hormonal-treated or radiation-treated cancer are negative for basal cell markers (p63, HMWK) and positive for alpha-methyl acyl-coenzyme A (CoA) AMACR (Figure 2-54).

■ Pancytokeratin immunostain may be a useful marker to highlight the neoplastic glands which are poorly formed and have cytoplasmic vacuolation.

■ PSA may be negative in some radiation-treated cancers.

DIFFERENTIAL DIAGNOSIS

■ Interpretation of posttreatment changes in benign and malignant glands in needle biopsies is a diagnostic challenge for pathologists.

■ For radiated-treated cancer, the differential diagnosis lies between prostate cancer with no treatment effect and benign prostatic glands with radiation changes.

■ Benign glands with radiation or hormonal changes may mimic prostate cancer.

■ For hormone-treated cancer, the differential diagnosis includes atrophic and hyperplastic changes in benign glands such as clear cell cribriform hyperplasia, sclerosing adenosis, atrophy, or post-atrophic changes.

■ Helpful features in the diagnosis of posttreatment prostate cancer includes an infiltrative appearance, blue mucin, intraluminal crystalloids, and presence of coexistent high-grade prostatic intraepithelial neoplasia.

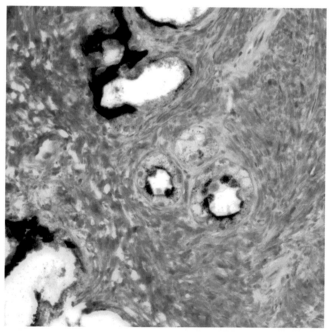

FIGURE 2-54

FIGURE 2-54 Prostate carcinoma with radiation therapy changes can still be positive for AMACR and negative for basal cells. A triple stain cocktail is helpful in confirming the presence of carcinoma with lack of basal cell staining and positive staining for AMACR.

Acinar Adenocarcinoma, Variant Differentiation

DEFINITION

■ Histological variants of prostate carcinoma comprise approximately 5% to 10% of prostatic carcinoma and are often seen concurrently with acinar prostatic adenocarcinoma. The histological variants differ widely in appearance and clinical behavior and include tumors with wide spectrum of morphological appearances such as foamy gland carcinoma and signet ring cell variants.

CLINICAL FEATURES

■ Histological variant of prostate adenocarcinoma include tumors that are different in terms of their clinical behavior with some tumors which are very aggressive such as small cell carcinoma.

MICROSCOPIC FEATURES

■ Foamy gland variant—An uncommon morphologically variant of prostate cancer with characteristic abundant foamy cytoplasm.
  ❏ Abundant foamy appearing cytoplasm with a low nuclear to cytoplasmic ratio (Figures 2-55 and 2-56).
  ❏ Cytoplasm is voluminous.
  ❏ Cytoplasm does not contain lipids but empty vacuoles (Figure 2-57).
  ❏ More typical features such as prominent nucleoli and nuclear enlargement are less pronounced (Figure 2-57).

(text continued on page 112)

Acinar Adenocarcinoma, Variant Differentiation (continued)

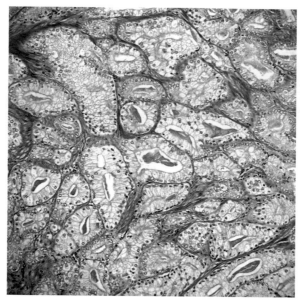

FIGURE 2-55

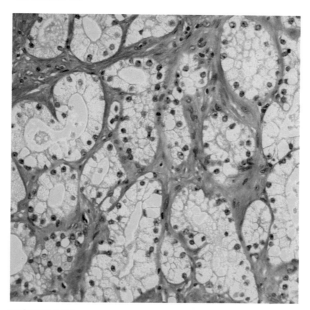

FIGURE 2-56

FIGURE 2-55   Foamy gland carcinoma with voluminous cytoplasm. Some of the glands contain pink secretions.

FIGURE 2-56   Foamy gland carcinoma with more bland cytological features and only a few scattered nucleoli visible at this magnification. Some of the malignant glands contain eosinophilic secretions.

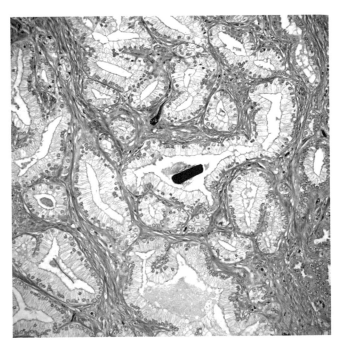

FIGURE 2-57

FIGURE 2-57   Foamy gland carcinoma with malignant glands with an infiltrative appearance. Note the presence of crystalloids and eosinophilic secretions within the lumen making these stand out from more benign glands.

Chapter 2: Premalignant Conditions and Prostate Carcinoma   *111*

Acinar Adenocarcinoma, Variant Differentiation *(continued)*

❏ In most cases, seen in association with ordinary adenocarcinoma of the prostate (Figure 2-58).
❏ Positive for PSA and PSAP.
❏ Negative for basal cell markers.
❏ Positive for AMACR.
❏ Differential diagnosis:
  • Benign crowded glands: Benign glands can sometimes mimic foamy cancer. However, the cytoplasm is more abundant in foamy cancer as compared to benign glands. Also, foamy cancer tends to have pink secretions in the lumen as compared to benign glands.
  • Mucinous metaplasia: This is a benign mimicker of foamy cancer. However, this type of metaplasia tends to be more focal and lobular as compared to foamy cancer. The glands are lined by rounded cells with goblet type cells. Furthermore, foamy cancer has more open lumen with pink secretions.
  • Cowper glands: In a needle biopsy, Cowper glands may mimic foamy cancer. However, Cowper glands are extra prostatic and present in skeletal type muscle. Also, Cowper gland usually has ducts and glands making it easier to recognize.
■ Atrophic variant—A distinct variant of prostate cancer, which has scant atrophic carcinoma and is often mistaken for atrophic glands.
❏ Resembles benign atrophy owing to its scant cytoplasm (Figure 2-59).
❏ Ordinary prostate carcinoma may become atrophic due to therapy effect but the atrophic variant does not have any prior therapy history.

(text continued on page 114)

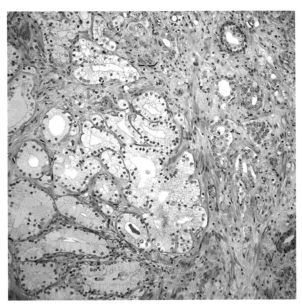

FIGURE 2-58

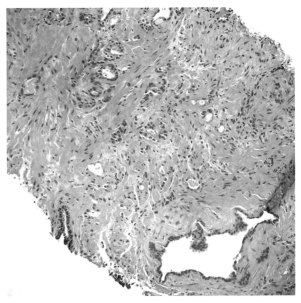

FIGURE 2-59

FIGURE 2-58   Foamy gland carcinoma with abundant cytoplasm with adjacent acinar carcinoma (usual variant) with more amphophilic cytoplasm.

FIGURE 2-59   Prostatic adenocarcinoma with mixed atrophic (bottom right) and usual variants (top left). Note the darker amphophilic cytoplasm of the nonatrophic usual variant adjacent to the atrophic variant. The infiltrative appearance of the atrophic variant and the merging of the atrophic cancer glands with the usual variant makes the diagnosis of atrophic cancer much easier.

Acinar Adenocarcinoma, Variant Differentiation (*continued*)

❏ Glands have a distorted lumen and somewhat flat appearance.
❏ Although atrophic, features such as prominent nucleoli and nuclear enlargement are present (Figures 2-60 and 2-61).
❏ Tumors usually have an infiltrative appearance and may be present adjacent to benign atrophic glands (Figure 2-62).
❏ In most cases, seen in association with the usual acinar adenocarcinoma of the prostate.
❏ Positive for PSA and PSAP.
❏ Negative for basal cell markers.
❏ Positive for AMACR.
❏ Differential diagnosis:
- Benign atrophic glands may appear to have nucleoli, particularly when evaluated at higher magnification. In the absence of architectural pattern of infiltrative glands, caution must be exercised in making a diagnosis of atrophic prostate cancer.

(*text continued on page 116*)

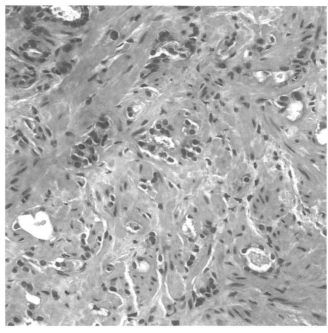

FIGURE 2-60

FIGURE 2-60 Atrophic variant of prostate cancer with glands which have crushed or distorted lumen and scant atrophic cytoplasm.

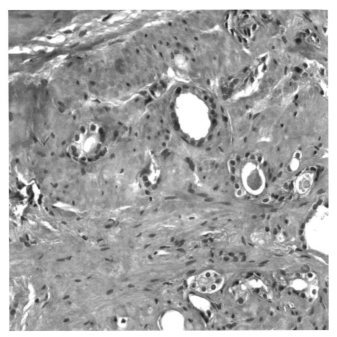

FIGURE 2-61

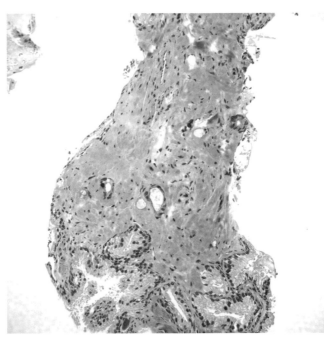

FIGURE 2-62

FIGURE 2-61   Atrophic prostate adenocarcinoma with an infiltrative appearance with significant
cytological atypia, including prominent nucleoli.

FIGURE 2-62   Atrophic prostatic adenocarcinoma with neoplastic glands infiltrating on both sides of
benign glands.

Acinar Adenocarcinoma, Variant Differentiation *(continued)*

■ Pseudohyperplastic variant—a distinct variant of prostatic adenocarcinoma that is characterized by the presence of larger benign-appearing glands with papillary infoldings.

❑ Resembles benign prostate glands in that the neoplastic glands are large with branching and papillary infolding (Figure 2-63).

❑ Numerous large glands with back-to-back straight luminal borders, and abundant cytoplasm.

❑ Significant cytological atypia may be present.

❑ Differential diagnosis includes high-grade prostatic intraepithelial neoplasia (HGPIN); basal cell markers are negative and AMACR is strongly positive (Figure 2-64).

❑ May behave aggressively with an extra prostatic extension.

❑ Usual Gleason score is 3 + 3 = 6.

❑ Positive for PSA and PSAP.

❑ Negative for basal cell markers (Figure 2-65).

❑ Positive for AMACR (Figure 2-65).

❑ Differential diagnosis:

• HGPIN may be mistaken for the pseudohyperplastic variant. However, HGPIN has basal cells.

• Benign hyperplastic glands can be mistaken for pseudohyperplastic variant of prostate cancer. However, they tend to have no cytological atypia and also have basal cells.

(text continued on page 118)

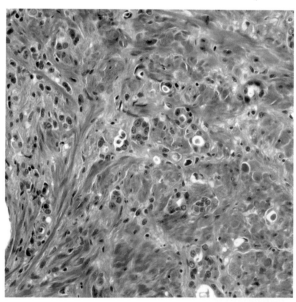

FIGURE 2-63

FIGURE 2-63   Atrophic prostatic adenocarcinoma shown at a higher magnification. Note the significant amphophilia and pronounced cytological atypia with prominent nucleoli and nuclear enlargement.

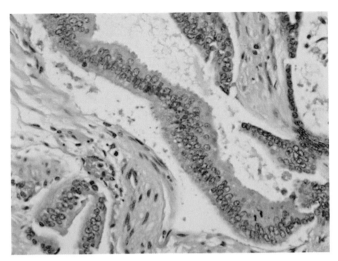

FIGURE 2-64

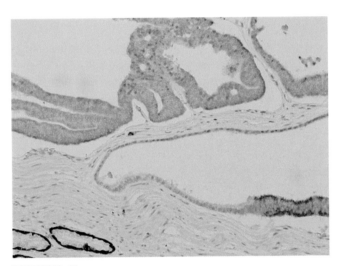

FIGURE 2-65

FIGURE 2-64 Prostate adenocarcinoma, pseudohyperplastic variant with glands with papillary infoldings. Note the cytological atypia and nuclear stratification, mimicking the appearance of HGPIN.

FIGURE 2-65 Prostate adenocarcinoma, pseudohyperplastic variant. Note the complete absence of basal cells as highlighted by negative basal cell markers (p63, HMWK) and positive AMACR staining.

Acinar Adenocarcinoma, Variant Differentiation (*continued*)

■ Mucinous (colloid) adenocarcinoma variant—A distinct variant of prostatic adenocarcinoma. Diagnosis of mucinous carcinoma should be made when at least 25% of the tumor resected contains lakes of mucin.
  ❏ One of the least common morphological variant.
  ❏ Diagnosis of mucinous cannot be made on prostate needle biopsy and if mucinous component is seen on a needle biopsy, it should be called prostatic adenocarcinoma with mucinous differentiation.
  ❏ Grossly, tumor nodules with mucinous and gelatinous texture may be seen.
  ❏ Single cells (Gleason pattern 3) or complex cribriform glands (Gleason pattern 4) are present, often in association with mucin pools (Figures 2-66 and 2-67).
  ❏ Usually seen in association with the usual variant of prostate adenocarcinoma.
  ❏ Behaves the same as the usual variant of prostate cancer.
  ❏ Positive for PSA and PSAP.
  ❏ Negative for basal cell markers.
  ❏ Positive for AMACR.
  ❏ Differential diagnosis:
    • Mucinous adenocarcinoma arising from the colon and involving the prostate. Immunohistochemistry will be helpful as the colonic adenocarcinoma will be CK20 and CDX positive while prostatic adenocarcinoma will be PSA and PSAP positive.
    • Mucinous adenocarcinoma arising from the urinary bladder or urachus involving the prostate. Immunohistochemistry may be helpful as the bladder adenocarcinoma will be CK20, thrombomodulin, and GATA3 positive while prostatic adenocarcinoma will be PSA and PSAP positive.

(*text continued on page 120*)

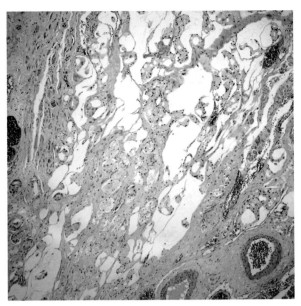

FIGURE 2-66

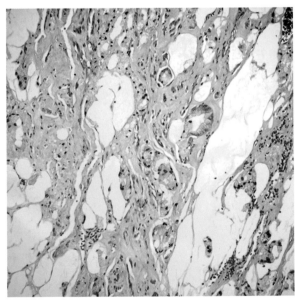

FIGURE 2-67

FIGURE 2-66 Prostatic adenocarcinoma, mucinous variant. Note the well-formed Gleason pattern 3 and some more complex Gleason pattern 4 glands are seen in intimate association with the mucin. Also note the presence of the adjacent usual variant of acinar adenocarcinoma.

FIGURE 2-67 Prostatic adenocarcinoma, mucinous variant. Note the Gleason pattern 3 glands which are well-formed. The glands have similar cytological atypia as the usual variant of prostate adenocarcinoma.

Acinar Adenocarcinoma, Variant Differentiation (*continued*)

■ Signet ring cell variant—A rare variant carcinoma of the prostate which is usually very aggressive and is characterized by the presence of an intracytoplasmic vacuole that compresses the nucleus into a crescent shape giving the appearance of a signet ring. It can occur in primary and secondary forms.

   ❒ Mean age at diagnosis is 68 years with ages ranging from 50 to 85 years.
   ❒ Some studies have suggested that malignant signet cells should constitute more than 20% to 50% of the tumor.
   ❒ Most often the signet ring cell pattern is seen as a minor component of Gleason pattern 5 tumors.
   ❒ Tumor predominantly consists of infiltrating single "signet" ring cells, of high Gleason grade (Grade 5) (Figures 2-68 and 2-69).
   ❒ Must be distinguished from vacuolated cytoplasm which may be seen in lower Gleason grade tumors.
   ❒ Usually positive for PSA and PSAP.
   ❒ Negative for basal cell markers and positive for AMACR.
   ❒ Positive for mucicarmine and alcian blue.
   ❒ Differential diagnosis:
      • Granulomatous inflammation.
      • Low Gleason grade prostatic adenocarcinoma with vacuoles which impart an appearance of signet ring cells.
      • Metastatic signet ring cell carcinoma from other sites such as bladder and gastrointestinal tract.
      • The presence of a primary signet ring cell carcinoma of the prostate should be confirmed by negative findings on gastrointestinal workup, and a positive stain for PSA.

(*text continued on page 122*)

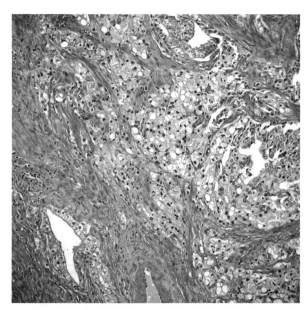

FIGURE 2-68

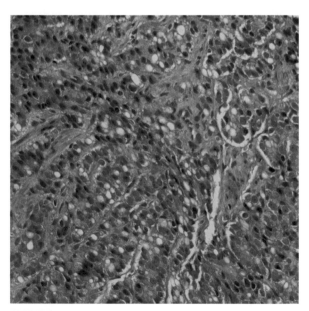

FIGURE 2-69

FIGURE 2-68   Prostatic adenocarcinoma, signet ring cell variant. The majority of the tumor (greater than 25%) consisted of signet ring type cells as shown here. The signet ring cells were PSA positive and there was no evidence of a gastrointestinal or bladder primary.

FIGURE 2-69   Prostatic adenocarcinoma, usual variant with prominent cytoplasmic vacuoles, giving the impression of a signet ring cell component in this prostatic adenocarcinoma.

Chapter 2: Premalignant Conditions and Prostate Carcinoma   *121*

Acinar Adenocarcinoma, Variant Differentiation *(continued)*

- Lymphoepithelioma-like variant—A rare histological variant of prostatic adenocarcinoma with a prominent lymphoid infiltrate admixed with malignant prostatic adenocarcinoma cells:
  - ❐ Clinical presentation includes elevated PSA and obstructive symptoms.
  - ❐ Characterized by syncytial pattern of malignant cells with a heavy lymphocytic infiltrate (Figures 2-70 and 2-71).
  - ❐ Prominent nucleoli and nuclear enlargement are present (Figure 2-72).
  - ❐ Malignant cells are PSA positive and cytokeratin positive.

(text continued on page 124)

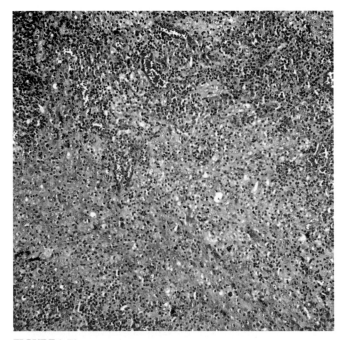

FIGURE 2-70

FIGURE 2-70   Lymphoepithelioma-like carcinoma of the prostate with a dense lymphocytic infiltrate almost obscuring the larger malignant cells with enlarged nuclei.

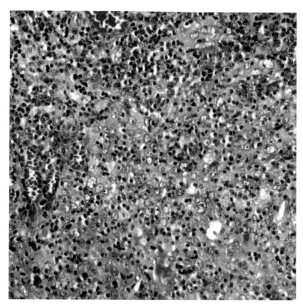

FIGURE 2-71

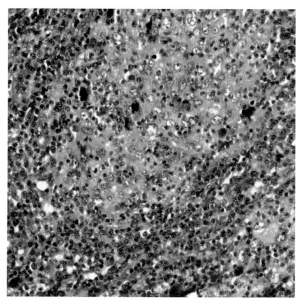

FIGURE 2-72

FIGURE 2-71   Lymphoepithelioma-like carcinoma of the prostate. Note the marked lymphocytic infiltrate admixed with the larger malignant cells.

FIGURE 2-72   Lymphoepithelioma-like carcinoma of the prostate. Note the presence of a more cohesive nest of malignant cells which are surrounded by a dense population of lymphocytes. The malignant cells have marked cytological atypia with enlarged nuclei and prominent nucleoli.

Acinar Adenocarcinoma, Variant
Differentiation *(continued)*

- ❐ The surrounding lymphocytes are predominantly T cells (Figure 2-73).
- ❐ Negative for Epstein-Barr virus by in situ hybridization.
- ❐ Differential diagnosis:
  - • Large cell lymphoma: The epithelial cells are strongly positive for cytokeratin making it easier to distinguish from a lymph proliferative process.
- ■ Sarcomatoid carcinoma—This is a rare neoplasm composed of both malignant epithelial and malignant mesenchymal elements.
  - ❐ This tumor may be composed of a varying mix of both malignant epithelial and malignant mesenchymal elements (Figures 2-74–2-76).
  - ❐ May have usual prostate carcinoma, usually higher grade, with varying amounts of nonspecific malignant spindle cell proliferation.
  - ❐ By immunohistochemistry, epithelial elements react with PSA and/or pancytokeratins.
  - ❐ Nodal and distant metastases are common.

(text continued on page 126)

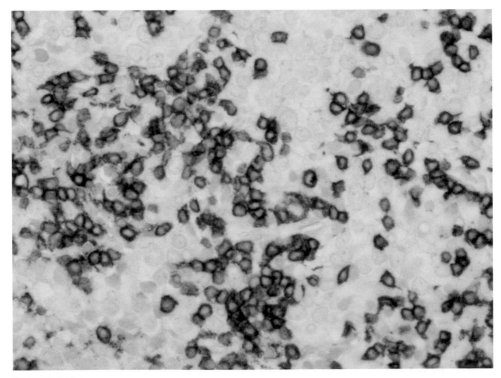

FIGURE 2-73

FIGURE 2-73 Lymphoepithelioma-like carcinoma of the prostate. A CD3 stain highlights the predominant population of T cells. A cytokeratin stain (not shown) will highlight the larger malignant cells.

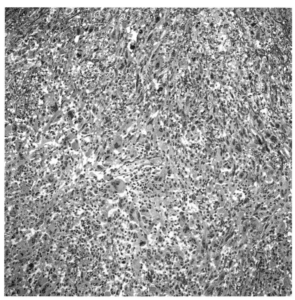

FIGURE 2-74

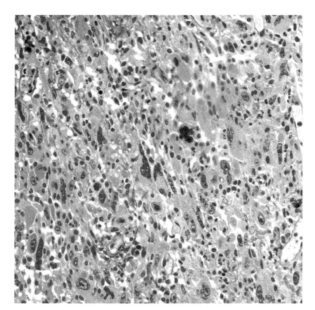

FIGURE 2-75

FIGURE 2-74 Sarcomatoid carcinoma of prostate highlighting a mixed population of epithelioid and spindle shaped cells with high-grade morphology, pleomorphism, and high mitotic activity.

FIGURE 2-75 Sarcomatoid carcinoma of the prostate with bizarre atypia and very little resemblance to an epithelial tumor. Majority of the tumor cells are undifferentiated and the lesion is indistinguishable from a high-grade sarcoma. A pankeratin stain is positive in this lesion (not shown here).

Chapter 2: Premalignant Conditions and Prostate Carcinoma   *125*

Acinar Adenocarcinoma, Variant Differentiation *(continued)*

❐ Differential diagnosis:
  • Primary prostatic sarcoma, including malignant phyllodes tumor, gastrointestinal stromal tumor, solitary fibrous tumor, or leiomyosarcoma.
  • Metastatic or direct extension of sarcoma or sarcomatoid carcinoma from urinary bladder or gastrointestinal tract.
▪ Pleomorphic giant cell carcinoma variant—This is a rare variant of prostatic adenocarcinoma which has characteristic pleomorphic giant cells with bizarre and anaplastic features.
  ❐ Conventional prostate cancer, even when very high grade, typically consists of cells with relatively uniform nuclei.
  ❐ In this variant, characteristic giant, bizarre, anaplastic cells are present.
  ❐ Marked atypia and presence of pleomorphic component ranges from 5% to up to 70%.

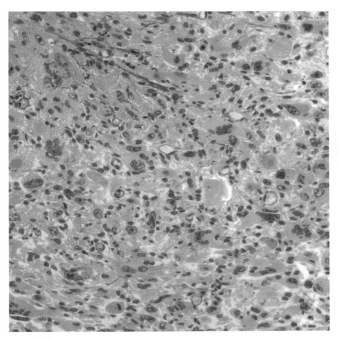

FIGURE 2-76

FIGURE 2-76   Sarcomatoid carcinoma of the prostate with marked atypia and high-grade features, including the presence of brisk mitotic activity with several atypical mitotic figures.

❐ Only a handful of cases with the prominent pleomorphism and bizarre giant cells have been described (Figures 2-77–2-79).

❐ This giant cell component is the hallmark of a particularly aggressive clinical outcome.

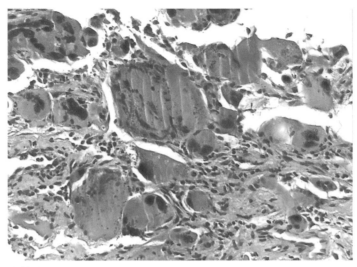

FIGURE 2-77

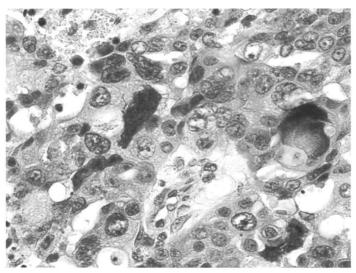

FIGURE 2-78

FIGURE 2-77   Pleomorphic giant cell carcinoma of the prostate. Note the presence of characteristic pleomorphic giant cells with bizarre atypia with abundant eosinophilic cytoplasm.

FIGURE 2-78   Pleomorphic giant cell carcinoma of the prostate with bizarre and pleomorphic cells admixed with an acinar component with fused malignant glands.

Chapter 2: Premalignant Conditions and Prostate Carcinoma   *127*

Acinar Adenocarcinoma, Variant Differentiation (*continued*)

- ❏ Differential diagnosis:
  - • Sarcomatoid carcinoma of the prostate, usually lacks the giant pleomorphic component.
  - • Radiation atypia in benign prostatic glands: The benign glands with radiation atypia usually have hyperchromatic nuclei but with a more degenerative type of atypia.
  - • Sarcomatoid carcinoma from other sites: Usually lack the pleomorphic giant cell component or may have rare cells with bizarre atypia. PSA should be negative in these tumors from other sites.
  - • Pleomorphic giant cell carcinoma originating in the urinary bladder and extending into the prostate: PSA and PSAP should be negative in these tumors. In addition, an in situ urothelial component may be present in association with the urinary bladder primary tumor.
- ■ Prostatic intraepithelial neoplasia (PIN)-like ductal adenocarcinoma—This is an uncommon variant of prostatic adenocarcinoma with pseudostratified columnar epithelium with papillary infolding and morphology resembling PIN.
  - ❏ Clinically, the patients present with elevated PSA or abnormal digital rectal exam, similar to the usual variant of prostatic adenocarcinoma.
  - ❏ The tumor is considered to be equivalent to a Gleason score 6 tumor unlike the ductal adenocarcinoma which is usually graded as 4 + 4 = 8.
  - ❏ Resembles HGPIN in terms of architecture (Figures 2-80 and 2-81).

(*text continued on page 130*)

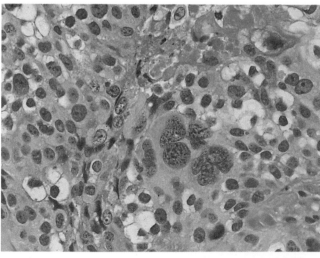

FIGURE 2-79

FIGURE 2-79   Pleomorphic giant cell carcinoma of the prostate. Low power showing the carcinoma with pleomorphic giant cells admixed with an acinar adenocarcinoma with perineural invasion.

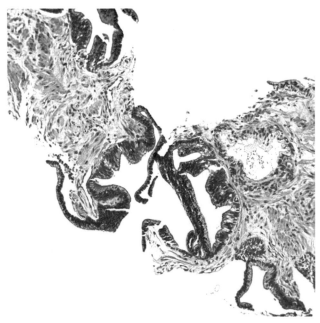

FIGURE 2-80

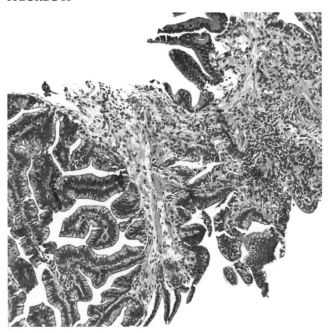

FIGURE 2-81

FIGURE 2-80   PIN-like ductal adenocarcinoma. Note the presence of glands with some tufting and some more flat glands, with an overall resemblance to HGPIN at low magnification.

FIGURE 2-81   PIN-like ductal adenocarcinoma. Note the epithelial lining which appears to be pseudostratified and columnar. The glands appear to be more crowded and have some architectural complexity of the ductal adenocarcinoma but still retain a PIN-like appearance.

Acinar Adenocarcinoma, Variant Differentiation (*continued*)

❑ The epithelium lining the neoplasm is similar to that seen in prostatic ductal adenocarcinoma with pseudostratified columnar cells (Figures 2-82 and 2-83).
❑ Positive for PSA and PSAP.
❑ Negative for basal cell markers.
❑ Positive for AMACR.
❑ Differential diagnosis:
  • HGPIN. PIN-like ductal carcinoma has an absence of basal cell markers (p63, HMWK) and is positive for AMACR, unlike HGPIN.
  • Prostatic ductal adenocarcinoma. PIN-like ductal carcinoma has less cytological atypia and architectural complexity and lacks the glandular and cribriform growth pattern. In addition, basal cell markers may show a patchy positivity in ductal adenocarcinomas.
  • Intraductal adenocarcinoma of the prostate. PIN-like ductal carcinoma has less cytological atypia and architectural complexity than an intraductal cancer and lacks the cribriform and proliferative growth pattern. In addition, basal cell markers may highlight the basal cells in the intraductal adenocarcinomas.

(*text continued on page 132*)

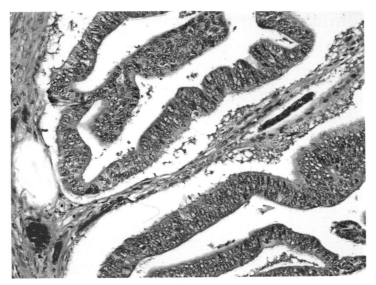

FIGURE 2-82

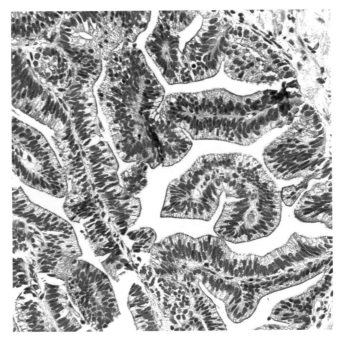

FIGURE 2-83

FIGURE 2-82   PIN-like ductal adenocarcinoma. Note the flat pseudostratified epithelium with columnar cells. Also prominent is the nuclear crowding and nuclear atypia.

FIGURE 2-83   PIN-like ductal adenocarcinoma. Note the presence of prominent small tufts of epithelium with some infolding mimicking a PIN lesion.

Chapter 2: Premalignant Conditions and Prostate Carcinoma   *131*

Acinar Adenocarcinoma, Variant Differentiation (continued)

ANCILLARY STUDIES

■ Basal cell markers (p63, HMWK) are negative while AMACR is strongly positive (Figure 2-84).

DIFFERENTIAL DIAGNOSIS

■ Differential diagnosis varies for each morphological variant.
  ❏ Foamy variant: Differential diagnosis includes Cowper's gland or mucinous metaplasia.
  ❏ Atrophic variant: Complete or simple atrophy.
  ❏ Pseudohyperplastic variant: PIN.
  ❏ Mucinous variant: Mucinous hyperplasia.

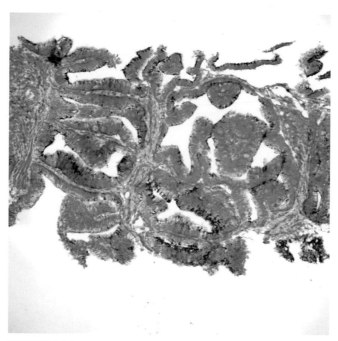

FIGURE 2-84

FIGURE 2-84   PIN-like ductal adenocarcinoma. A triple stain cocktail comprising of basal cell markers (p63, HMWK) and AMACR highlights the complete absence of basal cells with positive AMACR staining. This staining pattern is indistinguishable from that of the usual variant of prostatic adenocarcinoma.

Intraductal Carcinoma of the Prostate

DEFINITION
■ Intraductal carcinoma of the prostate (IDC-P) is a distinct entity which is characterized by the spread of prostatic adenocarcinoma into prostatic ducts or acini, most often seen in close association with invasive prostatic adenocarcinoma component.

CLINICAL FEATURES
■ Most patients have an elevated serum PSA.
■ Associated with high Gleason grade prostatic adenocarcinoma.
■ Commonly seen in radical prostatectomy specimens, particularly the ones with high volume disease.
■ Aggressive form of prostatic carcinoma.
■ Correlates with lesser progression-free survival and with increased postsurgical, biochemical recurrence.

MICROSCOPIC FEATURES
■ Cytologically atypical malignant cells fill the prostatic ducts and acini.
■ Expansion into the ducts may consist of solid, cribriform (typically densely packed), or micropapillary patterns (Figures 2-85, 2-86, 2-87, and 2-88).

(*text continued on page 136*)

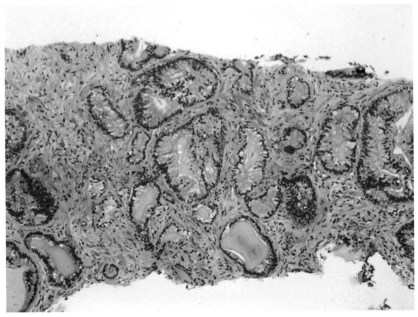

FIGURE 2-85

FIGURE 2-85 Intraductal and invasive prostatic adenocarcinoma involving a needle core biopsy. Note the small infiltrating adenocarcinoma seen adjacent to foci of solid or cribriform intraductal carcinoma.

Chapter 2: Premalignant Conditions and Prostate Carcinoma　　　*133*

Intraductal Carcinoma of the
Prostate (*continued*)

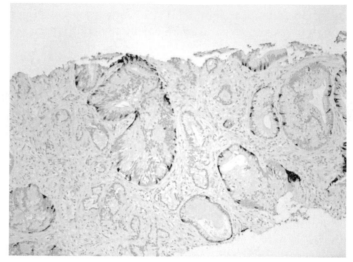

FIGURE 2-86

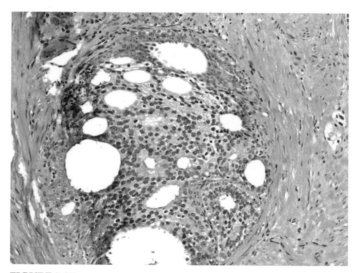

FIGURE 2-87

FIGURE 2-86 HMWK immunostaining of the case from Figure 2-85. Note the complete or patchy preservation of basal cells in the focus of the intraductal carcinoma with complete loss in the adjacent infiltrating adenocarcinoma glands.

FIGURE 2-87 Expansile proliferation of neoplastic glands within an existing prostatic ducts resulting in a dense cribriform pattern. The basal cells are apparent on the periphery of the lesion. Note the marked cytological atypia, including the presence of prominent central nucleoli.

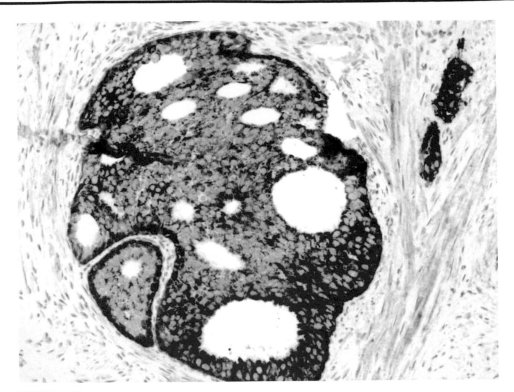

FIGURE 2-88

FIGURE 2-88   IDC-P (from Figure 2-87) as highlighted by the triple cocktail of basal cell markers (p63, HMWK, and AMACR). Note the complete preservation of basal cell layer highlighted by the basal cell markers with absent basal cell staining in the neoplastic cells expanding into the duct or invading into the adjacent prostatic parenchyma. The neoplastic cells within the ducts as well as the two invasive glands are highlighted by strong cytoplasmic AMACR staining.

Intraductal Carcinoma of the
Prostate *(continued)*

- Basal cells may be seen.
- Malignant cells typically have large, hyperchromatic, and pleomorphic nuclei with prominent nucleoli (Figure 2-89).
- Nuclear size of neoplastic cells is six times or larger than a nucleus from a benign duct (Figure 2-90).
- Comedonecrosis may be present in a subset of the cases.

ANCILLARY STUDIES
- Preserved or patchy basal cell staining with p63 or HMWK (Figure 2-91).
- Neoplastic cells with the ducts or acini are positive for AMACR and negative for basal cell markers (Figure 2-91).

(text continued on page 138)

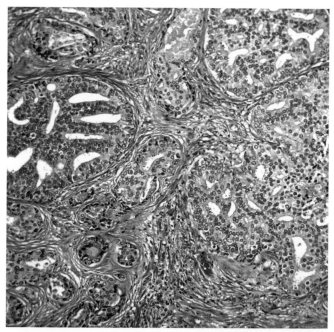

FIGURE 2-89

FIGURE 2-89   Intraductal and invasive prostatic adenocarcinoma involving a radical prostatectomy specimen. Note the small infiltrating adenocarcinoma seen adjacent to foci of solid or cribriform intraductal carcinoma.

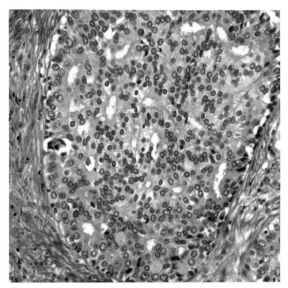

FIGURE 2-90

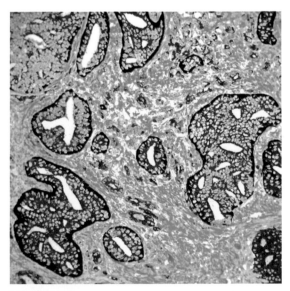

FIGURE 2-91

FIGURE 2-90   IDC-P. Note the solid expansile proliferation of neoplastic cells within the duct with marked cytological atypia including enlarged nuclei.

FIGURE 2-91   Cribriform pattern of IDC-P as highlighted by the triple cocktail of basal cell markers (p63, HMWK, and AMACR). Note the patchy or complete preservation of basal cell layer highlighted by the basal cell markers with absent basal cell staining in the neoplastic cells expanding into the duct or invading into the adjacent prostatic parenchyma. The neoplastic cells within the ducts as well as the surrounding invasive glands are highlighted by strong cytoplasmic AMACR staining.

Intraductal Carcinoma of the
Prostate *(continued)*

DIFFERENTIAL DIAGNOSIS

- Benign normal proliferations such as prostatic glands from central zone of the prostate or proliferative lesions such as clear cell cribriform hyperplasia or exuberant basal cell hyperplasia.
- High-grade prostatic intraepithelial neoplasia.
- Invasive cribriform acinar prostatic adenocarcinoma.
- Ductal prostatic adenocarcinoma (Figure 2-92).
- Metastatic adenocarcinoma such as from the colon.
- High-grade urothelial carcinoma either in situ extension into prostatic ducts or invasive into the prostatic parenchyma.

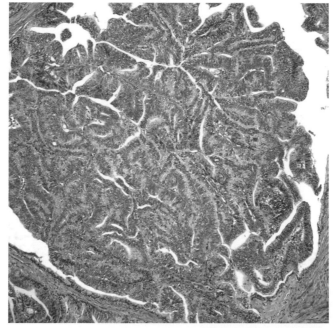

FIGURE 2-92

FIGURE 2-92   Ductal adenocarcinoma of the prostate. This lesion unlike intraductal carcinoma comprises of large ducts/acini filled with papillary or cribriform proliferation of neoplastic cells. The cells are columnar in appearance and have elongated nuclei. These lesions appear much more atypical than intraductal carcinoma with more pronounced cytological atypia, including the presence of prominent central nucleoli.

Prostatic Ductal Adenocarcinoma

DEFINITION
- Ductal adenocarcinoma (DAC) is a primary prostatic adenocarcinoma that comprises of large ducts/acini filled with papillary or cribriform proliferation of columnar cells.
- Also called adenocarcinoma with endometrioid features due to the distinct columnar cell morphology.

CLINICAL FEATURES
- Prevalence in prostatectomy and biopsy specimens ranges from 0.4% to 0.8% for pure DAC and up to 5% for mixed DAC and acinar.
- DAC is considered to be more aggressive and have a worse prognosis than prostatic acinar carcinoma.
- More likely to present with advanced stage cancer.
- Serum PSA is usually increased.

MICROSCOPIC FEATURES
- DAC occurs as either pure or, more commonly, mixed with acinar adenocarcinoma.
- Often seen in a periurethral location, but may also be seen in peripheral zones.
- Columnar, pseudostratified epithelium with abundant amphophilic cytoplasm, elongated nuclei, and prominent nucleoli (Figures 2-93–2-95).
- Papillary, glandular, or cribriform architecture (Figures 2-94 and 2-95).
- Slit-like cribriform lumen (Figures 2-96 and 2-97).

(text continued on page 142)

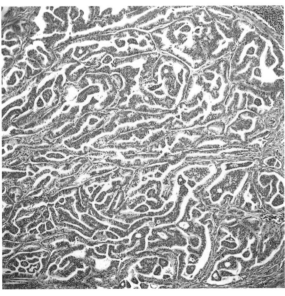

FIGURE 2-93

FIGURE 2-93   Prostatic ductal adenocarcinoma with prominent papillary architecture admixed with glandular architecture and amphophilic cytoplasm. Note the low power resemblance to endometrial carcinoma.

Prostatic Ductal Adenocarcinoma (*continued*)

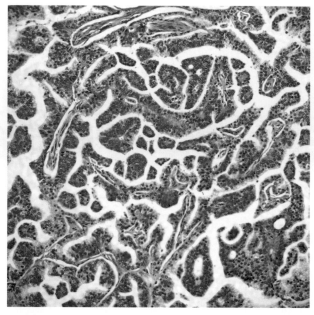

FIGURE 2-94

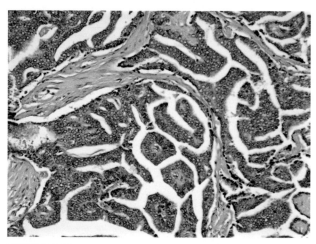

FIGURE 2-95

FIGURE 2-94 Prostatic ductal adenocarcinoma with pseudo stratification resembling high-grade prostatic intraepithelial neoplasia (HGPIN). Note the occasional slit-like spaces and the fibro vascular cores with tufting.

FIGURE 2-95 Prostatic ductal adenocarcinoma with marked cytological atypia, including hyperchromasia and prominent nucleoli. Note the nuclear crowding resulting in a pseudostratified appearance. The degree of atypia is far more than that can be seen in HGPIN.

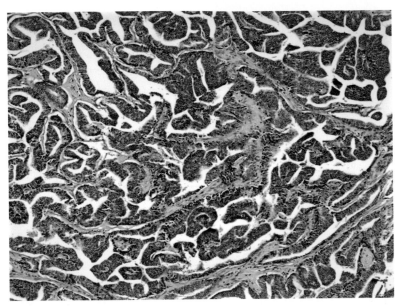

FIGURE 2-96

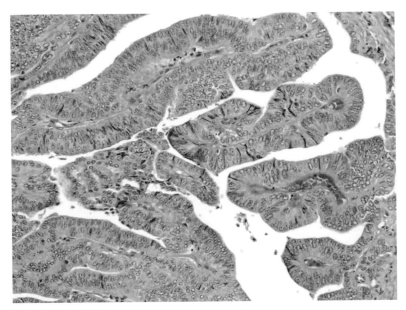

FIGURE 2-97

FIGURE 2-96 Prostatic ductal adenocarcinoma illustrating the complex cribriform structure with glandular appearance intermixed with prominent slit-like spaces.

FIGURE 2-97 Prostatic ductal adenocarcinoma with prominent papillary architecture, resembling HGPIN but with far more pronounced cytological atypia, including nucelomegaly and prominent nucleoli.

Prostatic Ductal Adenocarcinoma (*continued*)

■ Nucleomegaly (nuclear size: 2-3 times normal size) (Figures 2-97 and 2-98).
■ Mitotic figures and necrosis frequently present (Figures 2-99 and 2-100).

(*text continued on page 144*)

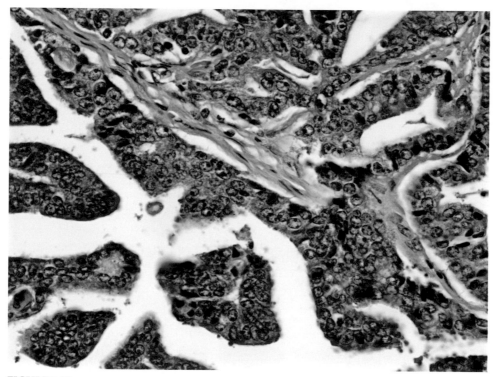

FIGURE 2-98

FIGURE 2-98   Prostatic ductal adenocarcinoma with marked cytological atypia, including nuclear hyperchromasia, pseudo stratification, and nuclear pleomorphism.

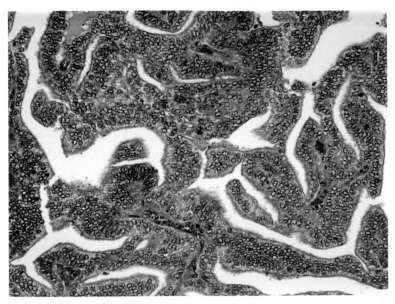

FIGURE 2-99

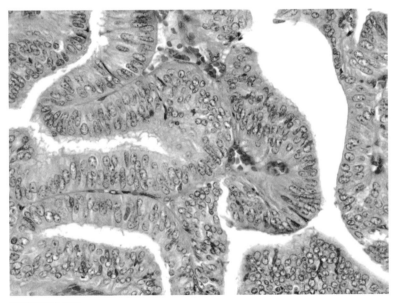

FIGURE 2-100

FIGURE 2-99   Prostatic ductal adenocarcinoma with complex cribriform architecture with marked cytological atypia. Note the nuclear crowding resulting in a pseudostratified appearance.

FIGURE 2-100   Prostatic ductal adenocarcinoma with pronounced pseudo stratification of the elongated nuclei. Note the marked nuclear atypia with prominent nucleoli and nuclear enlargement.

Prostatic Ductal Adenocarcinoma (continued)

ANCILLARY STUDIES
- Basal cell markers (p63, HMWK) are usually negative with rare patchy staining (Figure 2-101).
- AMACR (p504S) is strongly positive (Figure 2-101).
- PSA and PSAP immunostains are positive (Figure 2-102).

DIFFERENTIAL DIAGNOSIS
- Cribriform pattern of DAC may resemble HGPIN.
- Intraductal carcinoma of the prostate.
- Benign prostatic urethral polyp.
- Urothelial carcinoma.
- Metastatic colonic adenocarcinoma.

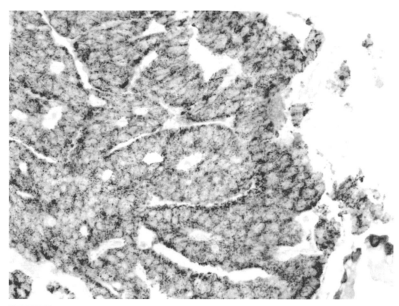

FIGURE 2-101

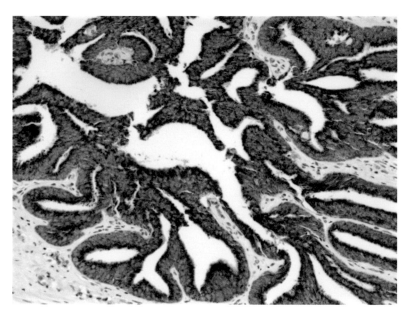

FIGURE 2-102

FIGURE 2-101 Prostatic ductal adenocarcinoma with strong staining with AMACR and absence of basal cell marker staining as seen in this triple cocktail stain (p63, HMWK, and AMACR). Note the prominent papillary and glandular architecture.

FIGURE 2-102 Prostatic ductal adenocarcinoma with strong staining for PSA. The latter immunostain is helpful in differentiating prostatic ductal adenocarcinoma from a metastatic colonic adenocarcinoma.

Small Cell Carcinoma

DEFINITION
- Rare histological subtype of prostate carcinoma (<1% of all prostatic cancers) which is high grade and with neuroendocrine differentiation.

CLINICAL FEATURES
- Adult males of older age (>60 years of age).
- May be associated with elevated PSA.
- Aggressive disease with poor prognosis with a median survival less than 1 year.
- Advanced stage at presentation.
- Similar therapeutic management as small cell carcinoma of the lung.

MICROSCOPIC FEATURES
- Microscopic features are similar to those seen in small cell carcinoma in other organs.
- Characteristic small neoplastic cells with minimal cytoplasm and with nuclear molding (Figures 2-103 and 2-104).

(text continued on page 148)

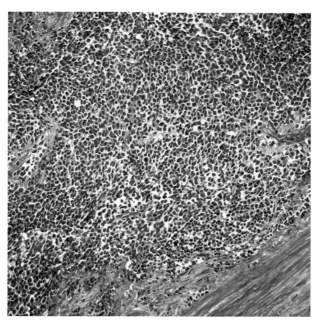

FIGURE 2-103

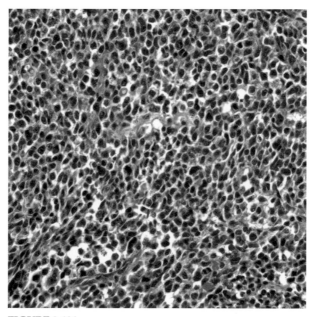

FIGURE 2-104

FIGURE 2-103   Small cell carcinoma within prostatic parenchyma with solid growth pattern and linear cords of neoplastic cells.

FIGURE 2-104   Small cell carcinoma with classic features such as a high nuclear to cytoplasmic ratio, indistinct nucleoli, and a suggestion of rosette formation.

Chapter 2: Premalignant Conditions and Prostate Carcinoma   *147*

Small Cell Carcinoma (*continued*)

- Chromatin pattern is fine (Figure 2-105).
- Rosette formation may be seen.
- Extensive tumor necrosis, apoptosis, *Karyorrhexis*, high mitotic rate (Figures 2-105 and 2-106).

ANCILLARY STUDIES
- Positive neuroendocrine markers.
- PSA and PSAP are either negative or only focally positive.
- CD44 is expressed in small cell carcinomas of the prostate but is rarely expressed in small cell carcinomas of other organs.
- TTF-1 may be positive.
- A subset of cases may be positive for TMPRS22-ERG fusion.

DIFFERENTIAL DIAGNOSIS
- Poorly differentiated prostatic adenocarcinoma (Gleason pattern 5). Typically, a Gleason grade 5 prostatic carcinoma will have more prominent nucleoli and more abundance of cytoplasm. A small cell carcinoma will have characteristic findings of high nuclear to cytoplasmic ratio, nuclear molding, and apoptosis as well as inconspicuous nucleoli.
- Metastatic small cell carcinoma from other sources such as the lung or urinary bladder.

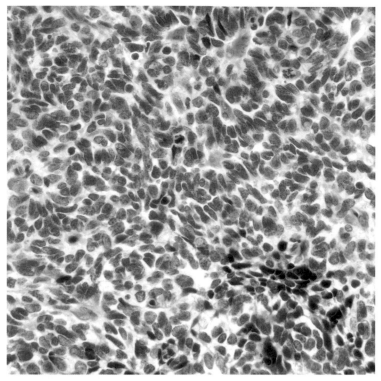

FIGURE 2-105

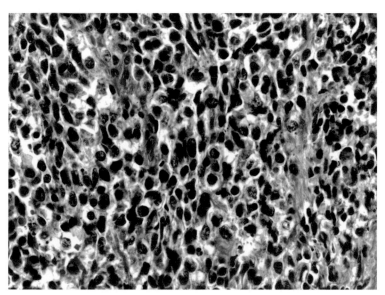

FIGURE 2-106

FIGURE 2-105   Small cell carcinoma with tumor cells growing in solid sheets with scant cytoplasm and a high nuclear to cytoplasmic ratio. Note the rosette formation.

FIGURE 2-106   Small cell carcinoma with high nuclear to cytoplasmic ratios, inconspicuous nucleoli, frequent mitosis, and apoptosis.

Chapter 2: Premalignant Conditions and Prostate Carcinoma   *149*

Prostate Carcinoma With Squamous Cell Differentiation

DEFINITION
- Prostate carcinoma with squamous differentiation is very rare and is often seen in cases with a prior history of radiation and/or hormonal therapy. These tumors are thought to originate from prostatic glandular cells.
- A secondary tumor involving the prostate from other sites must be excluded.
- Urothelial carcinoma with squamous differentiation must also be excluded.

CLINICAL FEATURES
- The age at diagnosis ranges from 49 to 86 years of age.
- Prostate carcinoma with squamous differentiation is usually associated with a poorer prognosis.
- Risk factors include prior history of adenocarcinoma, and/or radiation, or hormonal therapy.
- These patients typically have a poor response to surgical, hormonal, or radiation therapies.
- Metastatic disease in 30% to 40% of the cases.
- Serum PSA may be normal.

MICROSCOPIC FEATURES
- The squamous component may be the only component (100%, pure squamous cell carcinoma) or the squamous component may range from 5% to 95% (Figures 2-107, 2-108, 2-109, and 2-110).
- Pure squamous cell carcinoma is similar to squamous cell carcinoma from other sites such as the bladder, with infiltrating nests of malignant cells with abundant cytoplasm and intercellular bridges.
- Most common type of prostatic carcinoma with squamous differentiation is adenosquamous type with coexistence of glandular and squamous components with the adenocarcinoma component ranging from 5% to 95%, usually with a higher Gleason grade (Figures 2-111, 2-112, 2-113, and 2-114).
- Other components such as a sarcomatoid component may coexist with the squamous component.
- The degree of differentiation of the squamous component varies from well-differentiated to poorly differentiated, with varying degree of cytological atypia.

ANCILLARY STUDIES
- Prostate specific antigen (PSA) and prostatic specific acid phosphatase (PSAP) may be positive in the majority of the cases of adenosquamous carcinoma, confirming a prostatic origin.
- The squamous cell component may be PSA and PSAP negative and positive for HMWK.

DIFFERENTIAL DIAGNOSIS
- Squamous metaplasia with an adjacent infarct in the prostate. The degree of atypia in areas adjacent to an infarct may be very high.
- Secondary squamous cell carcinomas from other sites involving the prostate.
- Squamous cell metaplasia of benign glands with concurrent basal cell hyperplasia in patients treated with hormonal and/or radiation therapies.

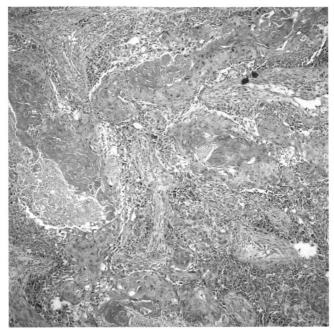

FIGURE 2-107

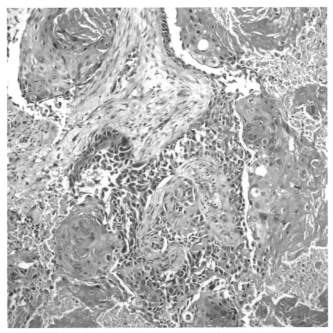

FIGURE 2-108

FIGURE 2-107 Prostatic carcinoma with squamous differentiation. This patient has a history of acinar adenocarcinoma of the prostate which was treated with radiation.

FIGURE 2-108 Prostatic carcinoma with squamous differentiation. Higher magnification of the case represented in Figure 2-107. Note the extensive keratinization.

(*continued*)

Chapter 2: Premalignant Conditions and Prostate Carcinoma   *151*

Prostate Carcinoma With Squamous Cell Differentiation (*continued*)

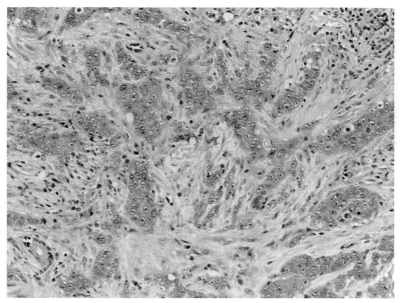

FIGURE 2-109

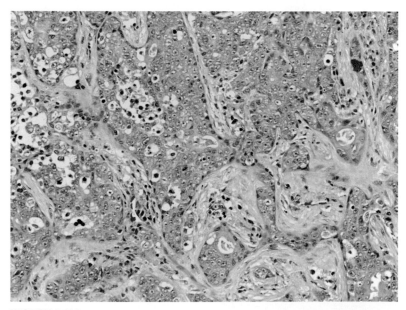

FIGURE 2-110

FIGURE 2-109 Prostatic carcinoma with adenosquamous differentiation. Note the squamous cell carcinoma component which is moderately differentiated. The squamous component is admixed with adenosquamous and acinar components. There is no history of radiation.

FIGURE 2-110 Prostatic carcinoma with adenosquamous differentiation. Note the scattered glands with both squamous features and suggestion of gland formation.

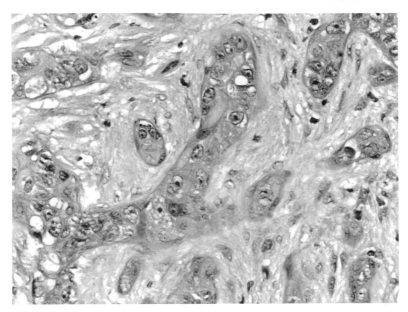

FIGURE 2-111

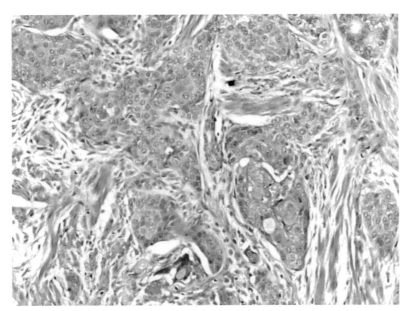

FIGURE 2-112

FIGURE 2-111   Prostatic carcinoma with squamous differentiation. Higher magnification demonstrating the eosinophilic cytoplasm and marked nuclear atypia.

FIGURE 2-112   Prostatic carcinoma with squamous differentiation. No glandular differentiation is seen.

(*continued*)

Chapter 2: Premalignant Conditions and Prostate Carcinoma   *153*

Prostate Carcinoma With Squamous Cell Differentiation *(continued)*

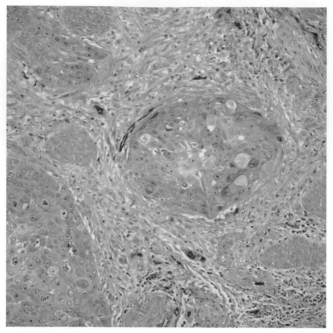

FIGURE 2-113

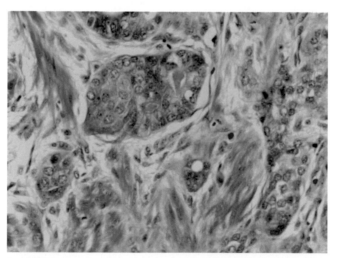

FIGURE 2-114

FIGURE 2-113   Moderately differentiated pure squamous cell carcinoma of the prostate from a patient with prior history of prostate carcinoma subject to radiation treatment.

FIGURE 2-114   Higher magnification of a focus of prostatic carcinoma with adenosquamous differentiation. Note the presence of gland formation intermixed with prominent squamous morphology.

Urothelial Carcinoma

DEFINITION
- Urothelial carcinoma involving the prostate may be primary or secondary.
- Primary urothelial carcinoma of the prostate arises from prostatic urethra, periurethral glands, and proximal prostatic ducts.
- Secondary urothelial carcinoma may involve the prostate either by growth of in situ urothelial carcinoma into prostatic ducts and acini (Tis) or by direct extension of an invasive urothelial carcinoma (T4).

CLINICAL FEATURES
- Primary urothelial carcinoma of the prostate is relatively rare, accounting for 1% to 4% of prostate carcinoma cases in adults.
- Secondary spread either direct or growth into prostatic ducts is more common and can be seen in up to 55% of cystoprostatectomy specimens from patients with invasive urothelial carcinomas.
- Age distribution is similar as in bladder urothelial carcinoma cases (45–90 years of age).
- Primary prostatic urothelial carcinoma patients typically present with obstructive urinary symptoms as well as occasionally with other symptoms such as hematuria and rectal pain.
- Serum PSA may be elevated.
- Prognosis depends on the status of invasion into the prostatic stroma.
- Survival rates are similar to bladder urothelial carcinoma patients.

MICROSCOPIC FEATURES
- Urothelial carcinoma in situ (CIS):
  - ❏ Urothelial carcinoma involves and completely fills the prostatic ducts and acini and may even extend into seminal vesicles (Figures 2-115, 2-116, and 2-117).
  - ❏ High-grade urothelial carcinoma shows marked cytoplasmic and nuclear atypia (Figure 2-117).
  - ❏ Occasional urothelial CIS may infiltrate into the surrounding prostatic stroma.

(text continued on page 158)

Urothelial Carcinoma (*continued*)

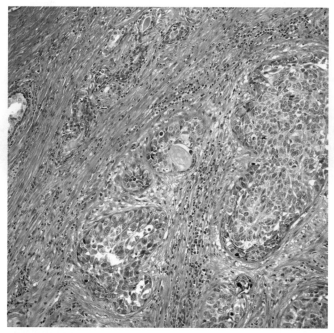

FIGURE 2-115

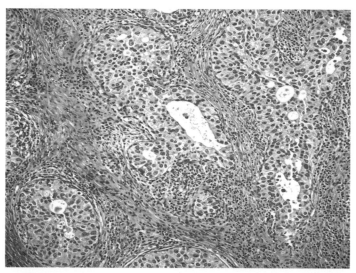

FIGURE 2-116

FIGURE 2-115   Urothelial CIS extending into prostatic ducts from a radical cystoprostatectomy specimen obtained from a patient with a large urinary bladder tumor involving the posterior and lateral wall. The tumor extends into perivesicular soft tissue but also grows into the prostatic ducts and acini.

FIGURE 2-116   Higher magnification of urothelial CIS (from Figure 2-115) extending into prostatic ducts. Note the prominent nuclear atypia, including pleomorphism and nucleomegaly.

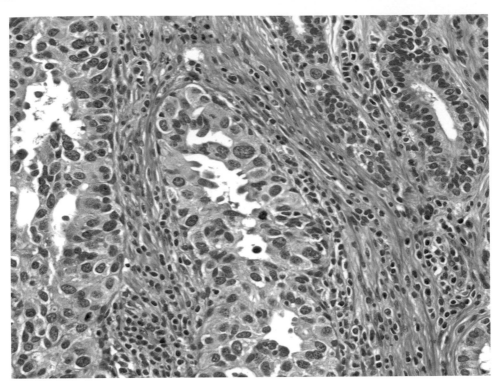

FIGURE 2-117

FIGURE 2-117 High power view of a prostatic duct involved by urothelial CIS. Note the absence of stromal invasion of urothelial carcinoma.

(continued)

Chapter 2: Premalignant Conditions and Prostate Carcinoma   *157*

Urothelial Carcinoma *(continued)*

■ Invasive urothelial carcinoma (Figures 2-118, 2-119, and 2-120):
  ❑ Invasive urothelial carcinoma may arise from CIS extending from a bladder primary urothelial carcinoma or from a primary urothelial carcinoma of the prostate.
  ❑ Usually stromal invasion leads to a striking desmoplastic response.
  ❑ The invasive component of the urothelial carcinoma may be very poorly differentiated (Figure 2-120).

(text continued on page 160)

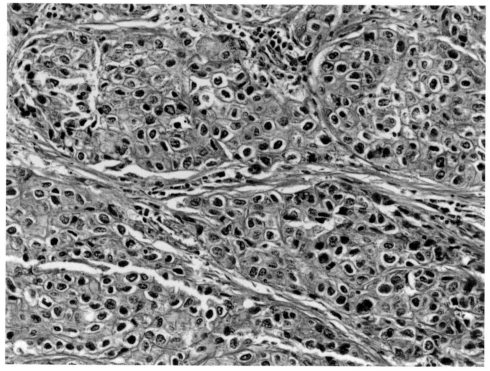

FIGURE 2-118

FIGURE 2-118   Invasive urothelial carcinoma arising from the urethra and extending into the prostate gland.

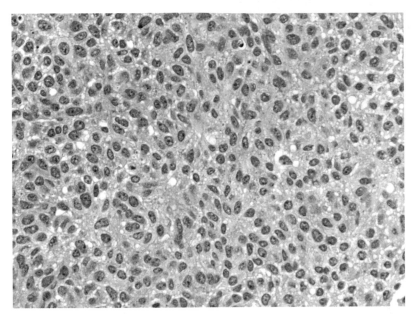

FIGURE 2-119

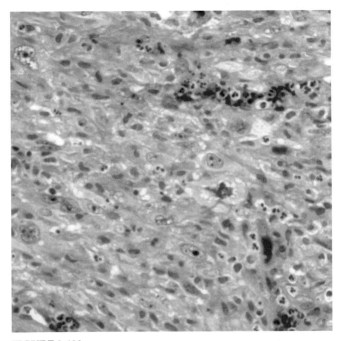

FIGURE 2-120

FIGURE 2-119   High-grade urothelial carcinoma involving the prostatic gland, most likely originating in the prostatic urethra. No carcinoma was identified in the urinary bladder from this patient.

FIGURE 2-120   Poorly differentiated high-grade urothelial carcinoma involving the prostate of likely urethral origin.

Urothelial Carcinoma *(continued)*

ANCILLARY STUDIES

- CK7 positive with variable CK20 staining.
- Usually positive for p63, thrombomodulin, GATA3, uroplakin, and HMWK (up to 65%–70% of the cases) (Figure 2-121).
- Prostatic markers such as PSA, PSAP, and P501s are negative.

DIFFERENTIAL DIAGNOSIS

- Poorly differentiated prostatic adenocarcinoma is often difficult to distinguish from a poorly differentiated urothelial adenocarcinoma, particularly in patients with a known bladder tumor (Figure 2-122). Prostatic origin may be confirmed by lack of basal cell markers (p63, HMWK) and strong AMACR staining (Figure 2-123).
- Intraductal carcinoma of the prostate may resemble intraductal or in situ urothelial carcinoma expanding into prostatic ducts. However, the intraductal carcinoma usually has a more complex architecture, including cribriform growth pattern. Prostatic origin may be confirmed by lack of basal cell markers (p63, HMWK) and strong AMACR staining.
- High-grade prostatic intraepithelial neoplasia.

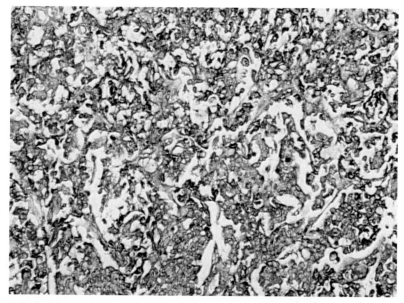

FIGURE 2-121

FIGURE 2-121 Poorly differentiated urothelial carcinoma, high grade highlighted by strong staining with thrombomodulin.

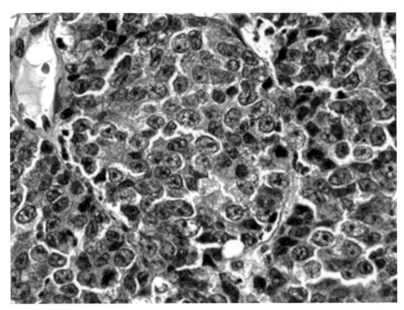

FIGURE 2-122

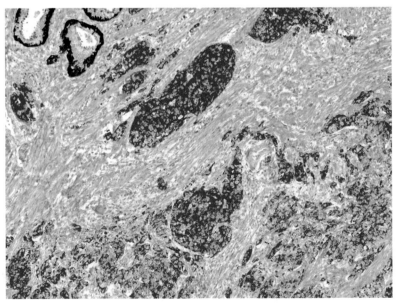

FIGURE 2-123

FIGURE 2-122 Poorly differentiated prostatic adenocarcinoma. This type of lesion is difficult to distinguish from a poorly differentiated urothelial adenocarcinoma, particularly in patients with a known bladder tumor.

FIGURE 2-123 Immunohistochemical staining to differentiate poorly differentiated prostatic carcinoma from an urothelial carcinoma. In this case, this is of prostatic origin as confirmed by lack of basal cell markers (p63, HMWK) and strong AMACR staining.

Mesenchymal, Hematopoietic, and Secondary Tumors

3

MESENCHYMAL TUMORS

HEMATOPOIETIC MALIGNANCIES

SECONDARY NONHEMATOPOIETIC TUMORS

Mesenchymal Tumors

DEFINITION
■ Primary or secondary spindle cell tumors involving the prostate.

CLINICAL FEATURES
■ These entities range from benign to aggressively malignant and present with clinical signs and symptoms that overlap with prostatic adenocarcinoma or benign prostatic hyperplasia, such as elevated serum prostate-specific antigen (PSA), abnormal digital rectal examination, and lower urinary outlet obstruction.

MICROSCOPIC FEATURES
■ Stromal tumor of uncertain malignant potential (STUMP) have hypercellular stroma containing atypical spindle cells. Nonneoplastic prostatic glands are admixed with the tumor. Leaf-like projections can be seen (Figure 3-1). The spindle cells have enlarged, degenerative appearing nuclei (Figure 3-2). The stromal projections are lined by normal appearing prostatic glandular epithelium. Areas of stroma that are hypocellular or myxoid can be seen. Mitotic figures are rare to absent and atypical mitotic figures should not be present. Blood vessels are not prominent.
■ Stromal sarcoma may occur independently or in conjunction with a STUMP. Tumors which exhibit overtly malignant stroma in which increased cellularity, cytologic atypia, necrosis, and/or mitotic figures are designated as stromal sarcomas instead of STUMP. Solid areas are more common than in STUMP, although leaf-like areas may be appreciated.
■ Leiomyoma will consist of well-formed fascicles, minimal cellular atypia, and rare to no mitotic figures.
■ Leiomyosarcoma is a tumor of smooth muscle in which mitotic activity, atypia, and hypercellularity are present. Necrosis may be seen.
■ Solitary fibrous tumor of the prostate is extremely rare and has morphology similar to other locations with a "patternless pattern" and thick, ropey collagen.

(text continued on page 166)

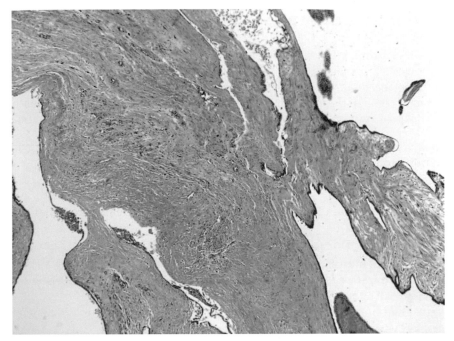

FIGURE 3-1

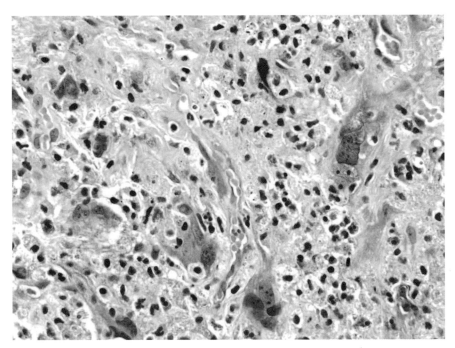

FIGURE 3-2

FIGURE 3-1   STUMP demonstrating leaf-like spaces and hypercellular stroma.

FIGURE 3-2   Markedly atypical stromal cells are present in this STUMP.

Chapter 3: Mesenchymal, Hematopoietic, and Secondary Tumors   *165*

Mesenchymal Tumors (*continued*)

- Gastrointestinal stromal tumor in this location usually arises from the rectum and only rarely invades the prostate. Spindle cells which are generally bland in appearance demonstrate a fascicular, palisading, or myxoid morphology (Figure 3-3).
- Rhabdomyosarcoma of the prostate is exceedingly rare and is usually of the embryonal subtype. Sheets of primitive cells in various stages of skeletal muscle differentiation are present.
- Inflammatory myofibroblastic tumor (postoperative spindle cell nodule) occur following procedures or prior instrumentation or *de novo*. These lesions consist of reactive fibroblasts, prominent small blood vessels, acute and chronic inflammation, and extravasated red blood cells.

ANCILLARY STUDIES

- STUMP is reactive for CD34 and progesterone receptor and usually expresses smooth muscle actin (SMA), muscle actin (HHF-35), and desmin (Figure 3-4). S-100, CD117 (c-kit), and anaplastic lymphoma kinase 1 (ALK-1) are negative. Stromal sarcomas have a similar expression pattern, although actin may show decreased expression.
- Leiomyoma and leiomyosarcoma express SMA, HHF-35, and desmin. Occasional expression of cytokeratin and progesterone receptor may be seen.
- Solitary fibrous tumor expresses CD34 and bcl-2 but is negative using AE1/3, S-100, and CD117 (c-kit).
- Gastrointestinal stromal tumor is positive for CD117 (c-kit) and CD34.
- Rhabdomyosarcoma is reactive for myogenin and myoD1. Typically SMA and desmin are positive while CD117 (c-kit) is negative.
- Inflammatory myofibroblastic tumor is usually positive for ALK-1, AE1/3, SMA, and desmin.

DIFFERENTIAL DIAGNOSIS

- Stromal nodule in benign prostatic hyperplasia: Stromal-only nodules in benign prostatic hyperplasia can mimic STUMP or leiomyoma. In contrast to leiomyoma, nodules in benign prostatic hyperplasia have numerous and prominent small stromal blood vessels. In contrast to STUMP, nodule formation by the stroma is present instead of atypical stromal cells interweaving through normal prostatic glands.
- Sarcomatoid prostatic carcinoma: A history of prostatic adenocarcinoma or areas of the tumor with gland formation are features to differentiate sarcomatoid carcinoma from malignant mesenchymal tumors. Ancillary immunohistochemistry, including PSA, prostate-specific acid phosphatase (PSAP), and broad spectrum cytokeratin (AE1/3) can be helpful.

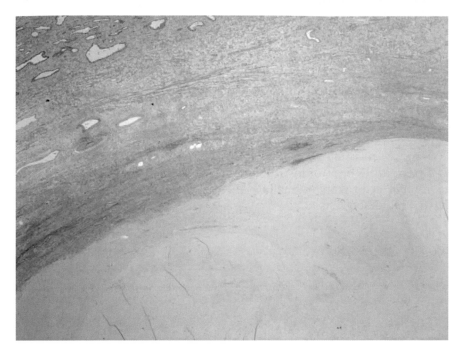

FIGURE 3-3

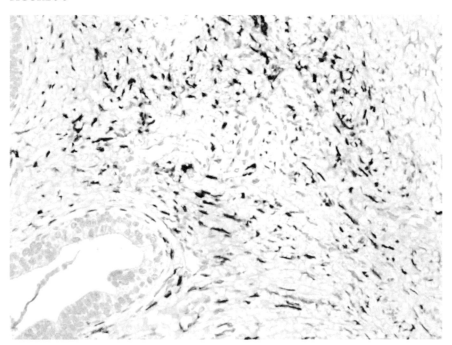

FIGURE 3-4

FIGURE 3-3   Gastrointestinal stromal tumor (bottom half of the photo) arising from the rectum with invasion into the prostate.

FIGURE 3-4   STUMP with progesterone receptor positivity. An adjacent nonneoplastic prostate gland is negative.

Hematopoietic Malignancies

DEFINITION
- Leukemia and lymphoma may rarely secondarily involve the prostate or pelvic lymph nodes resected with a prostatectomy while primary prostatic lymphoma is even more uncommon.

CLINICAL FEATURES
- The frequency of encountering a hematopoietic malignancy in a prostatectomy or associated lymph nodes is less than 1% of all cases.
- The majority of lymphoma involving the prostate is B cell lymphoma and very rarely Hodgkin's lymphoma.
- Incidental cases are detected at prostatectomy, including, most commonly, chronic lymphocytic leukemia/small lymphocytic lymphoma followed by marginal zone lymphoma and mantle cell lymphoma.
- Rare cases of nonchronic lymphocytic leukemia include monocytic, granulocytic, and lymphoblastic leukemia.
- Involved lymph nodes received with the prostatectomy are usually grossly enlarged.
- Presenting symptoms are due to lower urinary tract obstruction.

MICROSCOPIC FEATURES
- In chronic lymphocytic leukemia/small lymphocytic lymphoma, lymph nodes are diffusely effaced and the infiltrate in the prostate or lymph nodes is composed of small, monotonous, mature appearing lymphocytes (Figure 3-5). Pseudofollicle proliferation centers consisting of larger lymphoid cells are present (Figure 3-6). The infiltrate permeates the prostatic stroma, intervening between glands (Figure 3-7).
- Additional types of leukemia/lymphoma are less common and have features similar to that found at other locations (Figure 3-8).

ANCILLARY STUDIES
- Broad spectrum keratins such as AE1/3 are negative.
- PSA and PSAP are negative.
- CD45 is positive.
- Chronic lymphocytic leukemia/small lymphocytic lymphoma expresses CD5, CD20, bcl-2, and CD23 and is negative using CD3, CD10, bcl-6, and bcl-1.

DIFFERENTIAL DIAGNOSIS
- High-grade prostatic adenocarcinoma: High-grade prostatic adenocarcinoma may be composed of sheets of small cells that can mimic lymphoma. Areas of glandular differentiation are helpful in arriving at the correct diagnosis. In difficult cases, expression of broad spectrum keratin (AE1/3), prostate markers (PSA, PSAP), and negativity using hematopoietic/lymphoid markers (CD45, CD3, CD20) confirm the diagnosis of prostatic adenocarcinoma.
- Chronic inflammation: Chronic inflammation is typically periglandular and can involve glands and shows a mixture of lymphocytes and plasma cells, while a malignant lymphocytic infiltrate preserves glands and is homogeneous. Ancillary testing for aberrant expression of CD5 can be used to evaluate for chronic lymphocytic leukemia/small lymphocytic lymphoma.

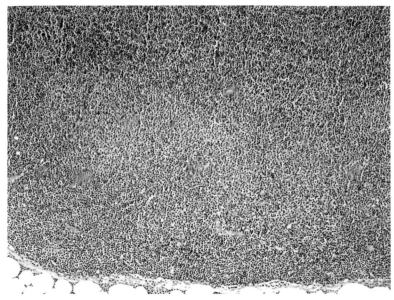

FIGURE 3-5

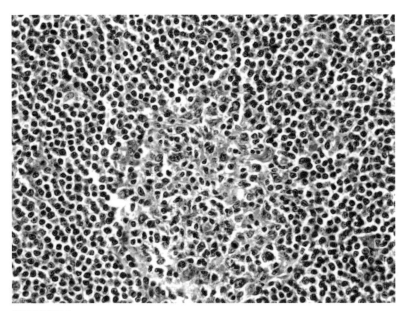

FIGURE 3-6

FIGURE 3-5   Chronic lymphocytic leukemia/small lymphocytic lymphoma involving a pelvic lymph node removed with a prostatectomy. The lymph node is effaced by a monotonous population of small lymphocytes.

FIGURE 3-6   In chronic lymphocytic leukemia/small lymphocytic lymphoma, pseudofollicle proliferation centers with larger lymphoid cells are surrounded by smaller lymphocytes.

(*continued*)

Hematopoietic Malignancies *(continued)*

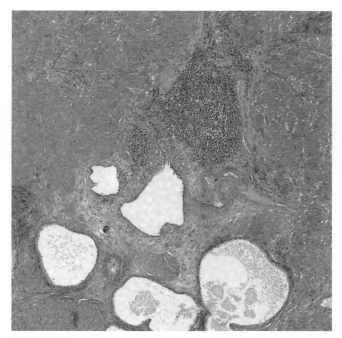

FIGURE 3-7

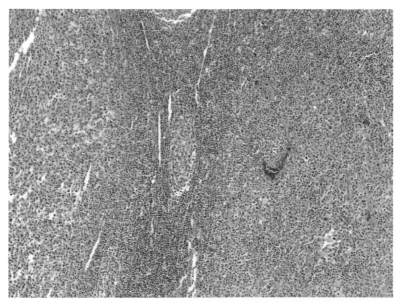

FIGURE 3-8

FIGURE 3-7 Chronic lymphocytic leukemia/small lymphocytic lymphoma involving the prostate. Note that the lymphocytic infiltrate does not have a periglandular predominance.

FIGURE 3-8 Follicular lymphoma involving a pelvic lymph node removed with a prostatectomy. Back to back neoplastic follicles are seen. Mantle zones are absent in the follicles.

Secondary Nonhematopoietic Tumors

DEFINITION
■ Nonhematopoietic tumors which involve the prostate by either direct extension or metastatic spread.

CLINICAL FEATURES
■ Tumors that spread by direct extension are usually from the bladder or colorectum.
■ Patients with metastases to the prostate typically have wide spread disease. Lung and the pancreas are the two most common sources.
■ A wide variety of other tumors have been described to occur in the prostate either by direct or indirect spread.

MICROSCOPIC FEATURES
■ Secondary bladder carcinoma involving the prostate can be intraductal or invasive. Intraductal tumors will have a nested appearance and intact basal cells surrounding the tumor. Invasive urothelial carcinoma may be rarely detected in needle core biopsies of the prostate (Figure 3-9). Plasmacytoid variant of urothelial carcinoma invades in single cells and chains of cells (Figure 3-10).
■ Colorectal carcinoma demonstrates glandular growth often with glands containing necrotic debris (Figure 3-11).
■ Lung and pancreatic adenocarcinoma can be encountered, demonstrating gland formation, and morphology similar to primary tumors (Figure 3-12).

ANCILLARY STUDIES
■ Urothelial carcinoma expresses CK7, p63, high molecular weight keratin (HMWK), and GATA3. CK20 may also be positive. PSA, PSAP, and alpha-methylacyl-CoA racemase (AMACR) are weak to negative.
■ Colorectal carcinoma is positive for CK20, CDX2, and beta-catenin (nuclear). CK7, PSA, PSAP, and AMACR are focal to negative.

DIFFERENTIAL DIAGNOSIS
■ High-grade prostatic adenocarcinoma with single cells: Urothelial carcinoma, particularly plasmacytoid variant, mimics high-grade prostatic adenocarcinoma that has a single cell growth pattern. Extensive tumor based outside the prostate favors a nonprostatic origin. Identification of areas with lower grade prostatic adenocarcinoma displaying well-formed glands is very helpful. Immunostains can confirm the origin.
■ High-grade prostatic adenocarcinoma with comedonecrosis: Colonic adenocarcinoma can mimic high-grade prostatic adenocarcinoma that has comedonecrosis. Glands consisting of tall, thin, columnar cells, hyperchromatic nuclei, and no macronuclei favor colonic adenocarcinoma. Immunohistochemistry may be used to differentiate these entities.

(continued)

Secondary Nonhematopoietic Tumors *(continued)*

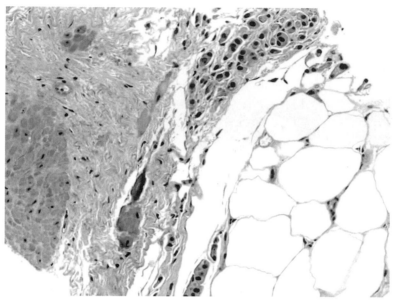

FIGURE 3-9

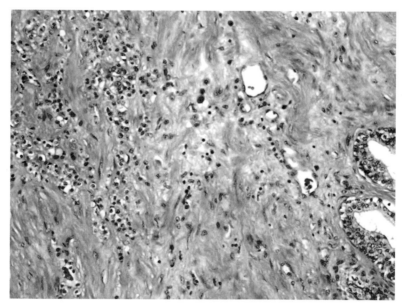

FIGURE 3-10

FIGURE 3-9   A needle core biopsy with unexpected urothelial carcinoma in the extraprostatic tissue.

FIGURE 3-10   Plasmacytoid urothelial carcinoma (left side of image) with single cells and chains of cells invading the prostate. Tumor cells have an appearance similar to plasma cells and lymphocytes. Two nonneoplastic prostate glands are present in the bottom right.

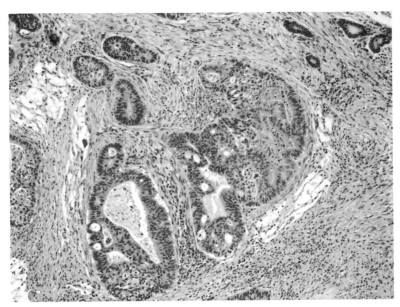

FIGURE 3-11

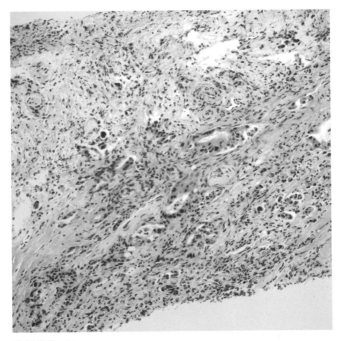

FIGURE 3-12

FIGURE 3-11   Direct extension of colorectal carcinoma into the prostate gland. Necrotic debris is present in the glandular lumens.

FIGURE 3-12   Pancreatic adenocarcinoma, with small glands and a marked desmoplastic stromal reaction, is identified in this prostate needle core biopsy.

Chapter 3: Mesenchymal, Hematopoietic, and Secondary Tumors   *173*

Bibliography

CHAPTER 1. NONNEOPLASTIC CONDITIONS

ACUTE INFLAMMATION

Hasui Y, Marutsuka K, Asada Y, Ide H, Nishi S, Osada Y. Relationship between serum prostate specific antigen and histological prostatitis in patients with benign prostatic hyperplasia. *Prostate*. 1994;25(2):91–96.

Nadler RB, Humphrey PA, Smith DS, Catalona WJ, Ratliff TL. Effect of inflammation and benign prostatic hyperplasia on elevated serum prostate specific antigen levels. *J Urol*. 1995;154(2 Pt 1):407–413.

Okada K, Kojima M, Naya Y, et al. Correlation of histological inflammation in needle biopsy specimens with serum prostate-specific antigen levels in men with negative biopsy for prostate cancer. *Urology*. 2000;55(6):892–898.

Ornstein DK, Smith DS, Humphrey PA, Catalona WJ. The effect of prostate volume, age, total prostate specific antigen level and acute inflammation on the percentage of free serum prostate specific antigen levels in men without clinically detectable prostate cancer. *J Urol*. 1998;159(4):1234–1237.

Roberts RO, Bergstralh EJ, Bass SE, Lieber MM, Jacobsen SJ. Prostatitis as a risk factor for prostate cancer. *Epidemiology*. 2004;15(1):93–99.

Rowe EW, Laniado ME, Walker MM, Anup P. Incidental acute prostatic inflammation is associated with a lower percentage of free prostate-specific antigen than other benign conditions of the prostate: a prospective screening study. *BJU Int*. 2006;97(5):1039–1042.

Schatteman PH, Hoekx L, Wyndaele JJ, Jeuris W, Van Marck E. Inflammation in prostate biopsies of men without prostatic malignancy or clinical prostatitis: correlation with total serum PSA and PSA density. *Eur Urol*. 2000;37(4):404–412.

CHRONIC INFLAMMATION

Anim JT, Udo C, John B. Characterisation of inflammatory cells in benign prostatic hyperplasia. *Acta Histochem*. 1998;100(4):439–449.

Delongchamps NB, de la Roza G, Chandan V, et al. Evaluation of prostatitis in autopsied prostates—is chronic inflammation more associated with benign prostatic hyperplasia or cancer? *J Urol*. 2008;179(5):1736–1740.

Platz EA, De Marzo AM. Epidemiology of inflammation and prostate cancer. *J Urol*. 2004;171(2 Pt 2):S36–S40.

Sciarra A, Di Silverio F, Salciccia S, Autran Gomez AM, Gentilucci A, Gentile V. Inflammation and chronic prostatic diseases: evidence for a link? *Eur Urol*. 2007;52(4):964–972.

Weidner W, Anderson RU. Evaluation of acute and chronic bacterial prostatitis and diagnostic management of chronic prostatitis/

chronic pelvic pain syndrome with special reference to infection/inflammation. *Int J Antimicrob Agents*. 2008;31 (Suppl 1):S91–S95.

GRANULOMATOUS INFLAMMATION

Agostinho AD, Corrêa LA, Amaro JL, Bacchi CE, Viana de Camargo JL. Malacoplakia or prostate cancer? Similarities and differences. *Urol Int*. 1998;61(1):47–49.

Furusato B, Koff S, McLeod DG, Sesterhenn IA. Sarcoidosis of the prostate. *J Clin Pathol*. 2007;60(3):325–326.

LaFontaine PD, Middleman BR, Graham SD Jr, Sanders WH. Incidence of granulomatous prostatitis and acid-fast bacilli after intravesical BCG therapy. *Urology*. 1997;49(3):363–366.

Oppenheimer JR, Kahane H, Epstein JI. Granulomatous prostatitis on needle biopsy. Arch *Pathol Lab Med*. 1997;121(7):724–729.

Sebo TJ, Bostwick DG, Farrow GM, Eble JN. Prostatic xanthoma: a mimic of prostatic adenocarcinoma. *Hum Pathol*. 1994;25(4):386–389.

Seo IY, Jeong HJ, Yun KJ, Rim JS. Granulomatous cryptococcal prostatitis diagnosed by transrectal biopsy. *Int J Urol*. 2006;13(5):638–639.

Tamsel S, Killi R, Ertan Y, Demirpolat G. A rare case of granulomatous prostatitis caused by Mycobacterium tuberculosis. *J Clin Ultrasound*. 2007;35(1):58–61.

Yurkanin JP, Ahmann F, Dalkin BL. Coccidioidomycosis of the prostate: a determination of incidence, report of 4 cases, and treatment recommendations. *J Infect*. 2006;52(1):e19–e25.

ATROPHY OVERVIEW

Billis A, Meirelles L, Freitas LL, Magna LA, Ferreira U. Does the type of prostatic atrophy influence the association of extent of atrophy in needle biopsies and serum prostate-specific antigen levels? *Urology*. 2009;74(5):1111–1115.

Billis A. Prostatic atrophy: an autopsy study of a histologic mimic of adenocarcinoma. *Mod Pathol*. 1998;11(1):47–54.

De Marzo AM, Platz EA, Epstein JI, et al. A working group classification of focal prostate atrophy lesions. *Am J Surg Pathol*. 2006;30(10):1281–1291.

Harik LR, O'Toole KM. Nonneoplastic lesions of the prostate and bladder. *Arch Pathol Lab Med*. 2012;136(7):721–734.

Kryvenko ON, Jankowski M, Chitale DA, et al. Inflammation and preneoplastic lesions in benign prostate as risk factors for prostate cancer. *Mod Pathol*. 2012;25(7):1023–1032.

Postma R, Schröder FH, van der Kwast TH. Atrophy in prostate needle biopsy cores and its relationship to prostate cancer incidence in screened men. *Urology*. 2005;65(4):745–749.

PARTIAL ATROPHY

Adley BP, Yang XJ. Alpha-methylacyl coenzyme A AMACR immunoreactivity in partial atrophy of the prostate. *Am J Clin Pathol*. 2006;126(6):849–855.

Brimo F, Epstein JI. Selected common diagnostic problems in urologic pathology: perspectives from a large consult service in genitourinary pathology. *Arch Pathol Lab Med*. 2012;136(4):360–371.

Herawi M, Parwani AV, Irie J, Epstein JI. Small glandular proliferations on needle biopsies: most common benign mimickers of prostatic adenocarcinoma sent in for expert second opinion. *Am J Surg Pathol*. 2005;29(7):874–880.

Oppenheimer JR, Wills ML, Epstein JI. Partial atrophy in prostate needle cores: another diagnostic pitfall for the surgical pathologist. *Am J Surg Pathol*. 1998;22(4):440–445.

Przybycin CG, Kunju LP, Wu AJ, Shah RB. Partial atrophy in prostate needle biopsies: a detailed analysis of its morphology, immunophenotype, and cellular kinetics. *Am J Surg Pathol*. 2008;32(1):58–64.

Wang W, Sun X, Epstein JI. Partial atrophy on prostate needle biopsy cores: a morphologic and immunohistochemical study. *Am J Surg Pathol*. 2008;32(6):851–7.

Worschech A, Meirelles L, Billis A. Expression of alpha-methylacyl coenzyme A AMACR in partial and complete focal atrophy on prostate needle biopsies. *Anal Quant Cytol Histol.* 2009;31(6):424–431.

OTHER TYPES OF ATROPHY
Billis A, Meirelles L, Freitas LL. Mergence of partial and complete atrophy in prostate needle biopsies: a morphologic and immunohistochemical study. *Virchows Arch.* 2010;456(6):689–694.

Brasil AA, Favaro WJ, Cagnon VH, Ferreira U, Billis A. Atrophy in specimens of radical prostatectomy: is there topographic relation to high-grade prostatic intraepithelial neoplasia or cancer? *Int Urol Nephrol.* 2011;43(2):397–403.

Sfanos KS, De Marzo AM. Prostate cancer and inflammation: the evidence. *Histopathology.* 2012;60(1):199–215.

ADENOSIS
Bostwick DG, Srigley J, Grignon D, et al. Atypical adenomatous hyperplasia of the prostate: morphologic criteria for its distinction from well-differentiated carcinoma. *Hum Pathol.* 1993;24(8):819–832.

Gaudin PB, Epstein JI. Adenosis of the prostate. Histologic features in transurethral resection specimens. *Am J Surg Pathol.* 1994;18(9):863–870.

Gaudin PB, Epstein JI. Adenosis of the prostate. Histologic features in needle biopsy specimens. *Am J Surg Pathol.* 1995;19(7):737–747.

Yang XJ, Wu CL, Woda BA, et al. Expression of AMACR (P504S) in atypical adenomatous hyperplasia of the prostate. *Am J Surg Pathol.* 2002;26(7):921–925.

BENIGN PROSTATIC HYPERPLASIA
McNeal JE. Origin and evolution of benign prostatic enlargement. *Invest Urol.* 1978;15(4):340–345.

Scattoni V, Raber M, Montorsi F, et al. Percent of free serum prostate-specific antigen and histological findings in patients undergoing open prostatectomy for benign prostatic hyperplasia. *Eur Urol.* 1999;36(6):621–630.

Van de Voorde WM, Oyen RH, Van Poppel HP, Wouters K, Baert LV, Lauweryns JM. Peripherally localized benign hyperplastic nodules of the prostate. *Mod Pathol.* 1995;8(1):46–50.

Viglione MP, Potter S, Partin AW, Lesniak MS, Epstein JI. Should the diagnosis of benign prostatic hyperplasia be made on prostate needle biopsy? *Hum Pathol.* 2002;33(8):796–800.

BASAL CELL HYPERPLASIA
Garcia FU, Haber MM, Chen X. Prostatic basal cells in the peripheral and transitional zones: zonal variation in morphology and in immunophenotype. *Prostate.* 2007 Nov 1;67(15):1686–1692.

Hosler GA, Epstein JI. Basal cell hyperplasia: an unusual diagnostic dilemma on prostate needle biopsies. *Hum Pathol.* 2005;36(5):480–485.

Rioux-Leclercq NC, Epstein JI. Unusual morphologic patterns of basal cell hyperplasia of the prostate. *Am J Surg Pathol.* 2002;26(2):237–243.

Thorson P, Swanson PE, Vollmer RT, Humphrey PA. Basal cell hyperplasia in the peripheral zone of the prostate. *Mod Pathol.* 2003;16(6):598–606.

Yang XJ, Tretiakova MS, Sengupta E, Gong C, Jiang Z. Florid basal cell hyperplasia of the prostate: a histological, ultrastructural, and immunohistochemical analysis. *Hum Pathol.* 2003;34(5):462–470.

Zhou M, Magi-Galluzzi C, Epstein JI. Prostate basal cell lesions can be negative for basal cell keratins: a diagnostic pitfall. *Anal Quant Cytol Histol.* 2006;28(3):125–129.

CLEAR CELL CRIBRIFORM HYPERPLASIA
Ayala AG, Srigley JR, Ro JY, Abdul-Karim FW, Johnson DE. Clear cell cribriform hyperplasia of prostate. Report of 10 cases. *Am J Surg Pathol.* 1986;10(10):665–671.

Frauenhoffer EE, Ro JY, el-Naggar AK, Ordóñez NG, Ayala AG. Clear cell cribriform hyperplasia of the prostate. Immunohistochemical and DNA flow cytometric study. *Am J Clin Pathol.* 1991;95(4):446–453.

TRANSITIONAL AND SQUAMOUS CELL METAPLASIA

Clark PE, Peereboom DM, Dreicer R, Levin HS, Clark SB, Klein EA. Phase II trial of neoadjuvant estramustine and etoposide plus radical prostatectomy for locally advanced prostate cancer. *Urology.* 2001;57(2):281–285.

Cowan DF, Orihuela E, Motamedi M, Pow-Sang M, Tbakhi A, LaHaye M. Histopathologic effects of laser radiation on the human prostate. *Mod Pathol.* 1995;8(7):716–721.

Gaudin PB, Zelefsky MJ, Leibel SA, Fuks Z, Reuter VE. Histopathologic effects of three-dimensional conformal external beam radiation therapy on benign and malignant prostate tissues. *Am J Surg Pathol.* 1999;23(9):1021–1031.

Guinan P, Didomenico D, Brown J, et al. The effect of androgen deprivation on malignant and benign prostate tissue. *Med Oncol.* 1997 Sep–Dec;14(3–4):145–152.

Lager DJ, Goeken JA, Kemp JD, Robinson RA. Squamous metaplasia of the prostate. An immunohistochemical study. *Am J Clin Pathol.* 1988;90(5):597–601.

Milord RA, Kahane H, Epstein JI. Infarct of the prostate gland: experience on needle biopsy specimens. *Am J Surg Pathol.* 2000;24(10):1378–1384.

MUCINOUS METAPLASIA

Bohman KD, Osunkoya AO. Mucin-producing tumors and tumor-like lesions involving the prostate: a comprehensive review. *Adv Anat Pathol.* 2012;19(6):374–387.

Gal R, Koren R, Nofech-Mozes S, Mukamel E, His Y, Zajdel L. Evaluation of mucinous metaplasia of the prostate gland by mucin histochemistry. *Br J Urol.* 1996;77(1):113–117.

Gaudin PB, Zelefsky MJ, Leibel SA, Fuks Z, Reuter VE. Histopathologic effects of three-dimensional conformal external beam radiation therapy on benign and malignant prostate tissues. *Am J Surg Pathol.* 1999;23(9):1021–1031.

Grignon DJ, O'Malley FP. Mucinous metaplasia in the prostate gland. *Am J Surg Pathol.* 1993;17(3):287–290.

Shiraishi T, Kusano I, Watanabe M, Yatani R, Liu PI. Mucous gland metaplasia of the prostate. *Am J Surg Pathol.* 1993;17(6):618–622.

NEPHROGENIC METAPLASIA

Allan CH, Epstein JI. Nephrogenic adenoma of the prostatic urethra: a mimicker of prostate adenocarcinoma. *Am J Surg Pathol.* 2001;25(6):802–808.

Harik LR, O'Toole KM. Nonneoplastic lesions of the prostate and bladder. *Arch Pathol Lab* Med. 2012;136(7):721–734.

Malpica A, Ro JY, Troncoso P, Ordóñez NG, Amin MB, Ayala AG. Nephrogenic adenoma of the prostatic urethra involving the prostate gland: a clinicopathologic and immunohistochemical study of eight cases. *Hum Pathol.* 1994;25(4):390–395.

Martin SA, Santa Cruz DJ. Adenomatoid metaplasia of prostatic urethra. *Am J Clin Pathol.* 1981;75(2):185–189.

Peeker R, Aldenborg F, Fall M. Nephrogenic adenoma—a study with special reference to clinical presentation. *Br J Urol.* 1997;80(4):539–542.

Xiao GQ, Burstein DE, Miller LK, Unger PD. Nephrogenic adenoma: immunohistochemical evaluation for its etiology and differentiation from prostatic adenocarcinoma. *Arch Pathol Lab Med.* 2006;130(6):805–810.

Young RH. Nephrogenic adenomas of the urethra involving the prostate gland: a report of two cases of a lesion that may be confused with prostatic adenocarcinoma. *Mod Pathol.* 1992;5(6):617–620.

RADIATION CHANGE IN NONNEOPLASTIC GLANDS

Brawer MK, Nagle RB, Pitts W, Freiha F, Gamble SL. Keratin immunoreactivity as an aid to the diagnosis of persistent adenocarcinoma in irradiated human prostates. *Cancer*. 1989 Feb 1;63(3):454–460.

Bostwick DG, Egbert BM, Fajardo LF. Radiation injury of the normal and neoplastic prostate. *Am J Surg Pathol*. 1982;6(6):541–551.

Cheng L, Cheville JC, Bostwick DG. Diagnosis of prostate cancer in needle biopsies after radiation therapy. *Am J Surg Pathol*. 1999;23(10):1173–1183.

Gaudin PB, Zelefsky MJ, Leibel SA, Fuks Z, Reuter VE. Histopathologic effects of three-dimensional conformal external beam radiation therapy on benign and malignant prostate tissues. *Am J Surg Pathol*. 1999;23(9):1021–1031.

Magi-Galluzzi C, Sanderson H, Epstein JI. Atypia in nonneoplastic prostate glands after radiotherapy for prostate cancer: duration of atypia and relation to type of radiotherapy. *Am J Surg Pathol*. 2003;27(2):206–212.

Martens MB, Keller JH. Routine immunohistochemical staining for HMWK 34-beta and AMACR (P504S) in postirradiation prostate biopsies. *Mod Pathol*. 2006;19(2):287–290.

Sheaff MT, Baithun SI. Effects of radiation on the normal prostate gland. *Histopathology*. 1997;30(4):341–348.

SEMINAL VESICLES/EJACULATORY DUCTS

Gaudin PB, Reuter VE. Benign mimics of prostatic adenocarcinoma on needle biopsy. *Anat Pathol*. 1997;(2):111–134.

Liu H, Shi J, Wilkerson M, Yang XJ, Lin F. Immunohistochemical evaluation of ERG expression in various benign and malignant tissues. *Ann Clin Lab Sci*. 2013;43(1):3–9.

López JI1, Angulo JC2. The ejaculatory ducts and their implications in prostate adenocarcinoma. *Anal Quant Cytol Histol*. 2013;35(4):205–209.

Quick CM, Gokden N, Sangoi AR, Brooks JD, McKenney JK. The distribution of PAX-2 immunoreactivity in the prostate gland, seminal vesicle, and ejaculatory duct: comparison with prostatic adenocarcinoma and discussion of prostatic zonal embryogenesis. *Hum Pathol*. 2010;41(8):1145–1149.

GANGLIA/PARAGANGLIA/PERIPHERAL NERVES

Ali TZ, Epstein JI. Perineural involvement by benign prostatic glands on needle biopsy. *Am J, Surg Pathol*. 2005;29(9):1159–1163.

Denford A, Vaughan M, Mayall F. Paraganglia as an unusual mimic of carcinoma in the prostate. *Br J Urol*. 1997;80(4):677–678.

Howarth SM, Griffiths DF, Varma M. Paraganglion of the prostate gland: an uncommon mimic of prostate cancer in needle biopsies. *Histopathology*. 2005;47(1):114–115.

Kawabata K. Paraganglion of the prostate in a needle biopsy: a potential diagnostic pitfall. *Arch Pathol Lab Med*. 1997;121(5):515–516.

Maniar KP, Unger PD, Samadi DB, Xiao GQ. Incidental prostatic paraganglia in radical prostatectomy specimens: a diagnostic pitfall. *Int J Surg Pathol*. 2011;19(6):772–774.

Ostrowski ML, Wheeler TM. Paraganglia of the prostate. Location, frequency, and differentiation from prostatic adenocarcinoma. *Am J Surg Pathol*. 1994;18(4):412–420.

Rode J, Bentley A, Parkinson C. Paraganglial cells of urinary bladder and prostate: potential diagnostic problem. *J Clin Pathol*. 1990;43(1):13–16.

Rossi G, Mengoli MC, Cadioli A, Cavazza A. Benign ganglion cells "invasion" in prostate needle biopsy. *Int J Surg Pathol*. 2012;20(3):260–261.

COWPER'S GLANDS (BULBOURETHRAL GLANDS)

Cina SJ, Silberman MA, Kahane H, Epstein JI. Diagnosis of Cowper's glands on prostate needle biopsy. *Am J Surg Pathol*. 1997;21(5):550–555.

Elgamal AA, Van de, Voorde W, Van Poppel H, Lauweryns J, Baert L. Immunohistochemical localization of prostate-specific markers within the accessory male sex glands of Cowper, Littre, and Morgagni. *Urology*. 1994;44(1):84–90.

Saboorian MH, Huffman H, Ashfaq R, Ayala AG, Ro JY. Distinguishing Cowper's glands from neoplastic and pseudoneoplastic lesions of prostate: immunohistochemical and ultrastructural studies. *Am J Surg Pathol*. 1997;21(9):1069–1074

COLONIC GLANDS

Hameed O, Humphrey PA. Pseudoneoplastic mimics of prostate and bladder carcinomas. *Arch Pathol Lab Med*. 2010;134(3):427–443.

Schowinsky JT, Epstein JI. Distorted rectal tissue on prostate needle biopsy: a mimicker of prostate cancer. *Am J Surg Pathol*. 2006;30(7):866–870.

CHAPTER 2. PREMALIGNANT CONDITIONS AND PROSTATE CARCINOMA

HIGH-GRADE PROSTATIC INTRAEPITHELIAL NEOPLASIA (HGPIN)

Bostwick DG, Qian J. High-grade prostatic intraepithelial neoplasia. *Mod. Pathol*. 2004;17(3):360–379.

Herawi M, Kahane H, Cavallo C, Epstein JI. Risk of prostate cancer on first re-biopsy within 1 year following a diagnosis of high grade prostatic intraepithelial neoplasia is related to the number of cores sampled. *J Urol*. 2006;175(1):121–124.

Godoy G, Taneja SS. Contemporary clinical management of isolated high-grade prostatic intraepithelial neoplasia. *Prostate Cancer Prostatic Dis*. 2008;11(1):20–31.

Eminaga O, Hinkelammert R, Abbas M, et al. High-Grade Prostatic Intraepithelial Neoplasia (HGPIN) and topographical distribution in 1,374 prostatectomy specimens: Existence of HGPIN near prostate cancer. Prostate. 2013;73(10):1115–22.

Montironi R, Mazzucchelli R, Lopez-Beltran A, Cheng L, Scarpelli M. Mechanisms of disease: high-grade prostatic intraepithelial neoplasia and other proposed preneoplastic lesions in the prostate. *Nat Clin Pract Urol*. 2007;4(6):321–332.

Zynger D and Yang X. High-grade Prostatic Intraepithelial Neoplasia of the Prostate: The Precursor Lesion of Prostate Cancer. *Int J Clin Exp Pathol*. 2009;(2):327–338.

FEATURES OF PROSTATIC ADENOCARCINOMA

American Cancer Society. *Cancer Facts & Figures 2013*. Atlanta, GA: American Cancer Society; 2013.

Brimo F, Epstein JI. Selected common diagnostic problems in urologic pathology: perspectives from a large consult service in genitourinary pathology. *Arch Pathol Lab Med*. 2012;136(4):360–371.

Epstein JI. An update of the Gleason grading system. *J Urol*. 2010;183:433–440.

Varma M, Lee MW, Tamboli P, et al. Morphologic criteria for the diagnosis of prostatic adenocarcinoma in needle biopsy specimens. A study of 250 consecutive cases in a routine surgical pathology practice. *Arch Pathol Lab Med*. 2002;126(5):554–561.

Zelefsky MJ, Eastham JA, Sartor OA. Cancer of the prostate. In: DeVita VT, Hellman S, Rosenberg SA, eds. *Cancer: Principles and Practice of Oncology*. 9th ed. Philadelphia, PA: Lippincott-Raven; 2011:1220–1271.

ATYPICAL SMALL ACINAR PROLIFERATION

Brimo F, Vollmer RT, Corcos J, Humphrey PA, Bismar TA. Outcome for repeated biopsy of the prostate: roles of serum PSA, small atypical glands, and prostatic intraepithelial neoplasia. *Am J Clin Pathol*. 2007;128(4):648–651.

Bostwick DG, Meiers I. Atypical small acinar proliferation in the prostate: clinical significance in 2006. *Arch Pathol Lab Med*. 2006;130(7):952–927.

Iczkowski KA. Current prostate biopsy interpretation: criteria for cancer, atypical small acinar proliferation, high-grade prostatic intraepithelial neoplasia, and use of immunostains. *Arch Pathol Lab Med*. 2006;130(6):835–843.

Strand CL, Aponte SL, Chatterjee M, et al. Improved resolution of diagnostic problems in selected prostate needle biopsy specimens by using the ASAP workup: a prospective study of interval sections vs new recut sections. *Am J Clin Pathol*. 2010;134(2):293–298.

Scattoni V, Raber M, Capitanio U, et al. The optimal rebiopsy prostatic scheme depends on patient clinical characteristics: results of a recursive partitioning analysis based on a 24-core systematic scheme. *Eur Urol*. 2011;60(4):834–841.

ACINAR ADENOCARCINOMA, GLEASON GRADING

Epstein JI. An update of the Gleason grading system. *J Urol*. 2010;183:433–440.

Epstein JI, Allsbrook WC, Jr, Amin MB, et al. The 2005 International Society of Urological Pathology (ISUP) Consensus Conference on Gleason Grading of Prostatic Carcinoma. *Am J Surg Pathol*. 2005;29:1228–1242.

Gleason DF. Histologic grading and clinical staging of prostatic carcinoma. In M. Tannenbaum, ed. *Urologic Pathology: The Prostate*. Philadelphia, PA: Lea and Febiger; 1977:171–198.

Gleason DF, Mellinger GT. Prediction of prognosis for prostatic adenocarcinoma by combined histological grading and clinical staging. *J Urol*. 1974;111:58–64.

Hattab EM, Koch MO, Eble JN, et al. Tertiary Gleason pattern 5 is a powerful predictor of biochemical relapse in patients with Gleason score 7 prostatic adenocarcinoma. *J Urol* 2006;175:1695–1699; discussion 1699.

Iczkowski KA, Bostwick DG. The pathologist as optimist: Cancer grade deflation in prostatic needle biopsies. Editorial. *Am J Surg Pathol*. 1998;22(10):1169–1170.

Poulos CK, Daggy JK, Cheng L. Preoperative prediction of Gleason grade in radical prostatectomy specimens: the influence of different Gleason grades from multiple positive biopsy sites. *Mod Pathol*. 2005;18:228–234.

Steinberg DM, Sauvageot J, Piantadosi S, et al. Correlation of prostate needle biopsy and radical prostatectomy Gleason grade in academic and community settings. *Am J Surg Pathol*. 1997;21:566–576.

ACINAR ADENOCARCINOMA, TREATMENT EFFECT

Armas OA, Aprikian AG, Melamed J, et al. Clinical and pathobiological effects of neoadjuvant total androgen ablation therapy on clinically localized prostatic adenocarcinoma. *Am J Surg Pathol*. 1994;18(10):979–991.

Bostwick DG, Meiers I. Diagnosis of prostatic carcinoma after therapy. *Arch Pathol Lab Med*. 2007;131(3):360–371.

Petraki CD, Sfikas CP. Histopathological changes induced by therapies in the benign prostate and prostate adenocarcinoma. *Histol Histopathol*. 2007;22(1):107–118.

Reuter VE. Pathological changes in benign and malignant prostatic tissue following androgen deprivation therapy. *Urology*. 1997;49 (Suppl 3A):16–22.

Rubin MA, Allory Y, Molinie V, et al. Effects of long-term finasteride treatment on prostate cancer morphology and clinical outcome. *Urology*. 2005;66(5):930–934.

Sung MT, Jiang Z, Montironi R, MacLennan GT, Mazzucchelli R, Cheng L. AMACR (P504S)/34betaE12/p63 triple cocktail stain in prostatic adenocarcinoma after hormonal therapy. *Hum Pathol*. 2007;38(2):332–341.

ACINAR ADENOCARCINOMA, VARIANT DIFFERENTIATION

Abbas F, Civantos F, Benedetto P, Soloway MS. Small cell carcinoma of the bladder and prostate. *Urology* 1995; 46: 617–630.

Alline KM, Cohen MB. Signet-ring cell carcinoma of the prostate. *Arch Pathol Lab Med*. 1992;116(1):99–102.

Epstein JH, Lieberman PH. Mucinous adenocarcinoma of the prostate gland. *Am J Surg Pathol* 1985;9(4): 299–308.

Hejka AG, England DM. Signet ring cell carcinoma of prostate: immunohistochemical and ultrastructural study of a case. *Urology*. 1989;34(3):155–158.

Hertell JD, Humphrey PA. Ductal adenocarcinoma of the prostate. *J Urol.* 2011;186:277–278.

Levi AW, Epstein JI. Pseudohyperplastic prostatic adenocarcinoma on needle biopsy and simple prostatectomy. *Am J Surg Pathol.* 2000;24(8):1039–1046.

Mazzucchelli R, Lopez-Beltran A, Cheng L, Scarpelli M, Kirkali Z, Montironi R. Rare and unusual histological variants of prostatic carcinoma: clinical significance. *BJU Int.* 2008;102:1369–1374.

Millar EK, Sharma NK, Lessels AM. Ductal (endometrioid) carcinoma of the prostate: a clinicopathological study of 16 cases. *Histopathology.* 1996;29:11–19.

Nelson RS, Epstein JI. Prostatic carcinoma with abundant xanthomatous cytoplasm: Foamy gland carcinoma. *Am J Surg Pathol.* 1996;20(4):419–426.

Oesterling JE, Hauzer CG, Farrow GM. Small cell anaplastic carcinoma of the prostate: A clinical, pathologic, and immunohistological study of 27 patients. *The Journal of Urology.* 1992;147:804–807.

Oliai BR, Kahane H, Epstein JI. A clinicopathologic analysis of urothelial carcinomas diagnosed on prostate needle biopsy. *Am J Surg Pathol.* 2001;25(6):794–801.

Osunkoya AO, Nielsen ME, Epstein JI. Prognosis of mucinous adenocarcinoma of the prostate treated by radical prostatectomy: a study of 47 cases. *Am J Surg Pathol.* 2008;32(3):468–472.

Parwani AV, Kronz JD, Genega EM, Gaudin P, Chang S, Epstein JI. Prostate carcinoma with squamous differentiation: an analysis of 33 cases. *Am J Surg Pathol.* 2004;(28)5:651–657.

Parwani AV, Herawi M and Epstein JI. Pleomorphic giant cell adenocarcinoma of the prostate: report of 6 cases. *Am J Surg Pathol.* 2006; 30(10):1254–1259

Randolph TL, Amin MB, Ro JY, Ayala AG. Histologic variants of adenocarcinoma and other carcinomas of the prostate: Pathologic criteria and clinical significance. *Mod Pathol.* 1997;10(6):612–629.

Spiess PE, Pettaway CA, Vakar-Lopez F, et al. Treatment outcomes of small cell carcinoma of the prostate: a single-center study. *Cancer.* 2007;110:1729–1737.

Warner JN, Nakamura LY, Pacelli A, Humphreys MR, Castle EP. Primary signet ring cell carcinoma of the prostate. *Mayo Clin Proc.* 2010;85:1130–1136.

INTRADUCTAL CARCINOMA OF THE PROSTATE

Cohen RJ, McNeal JE, Baillie T. Patterns of differentiation and proliferation in intraductal carcinoma of the prostate: significance for cancer progression. *Prostate.* 2000;43(1):11–19.

Cohen RJ, Wheeler TM, Bonkhoff H, Rubin MA. A proposal on the identification, histologic reporting, and implications of intraductal prostatic carcinoma. *Arch Pathol Lab Med.* 2007;131(7):1103–1109.

Guo CC, Epstein JI. Intraductal carcinoma of the prostate on needle biopsy: histologic features and clinical significance. *Mod Pathol.* 2006;19(12):1528–1535.

Han B, Suleman K, Wang L, et al. *ETS* gene aberrations in atypical cribriform lesions of the prostate: implications for the distinction between intraductal carcinoma of the prostate and cribriform high-grade prostatic intraepithelial neoplasia. *Am J Surg Pathol.* 2010;34(4):478–485.

Henry PC, Evans AJ. Intraductal carcinoma of the prostate: a distinct histopathological entity with important prognostic implications. *J Clin Pathol.* 2009;62(7):579–583.

McNeal JE, Yemoto CE. Spread of adenocarcinoma within prostatic ducts and acini: morphologic and clinical correlations. *Am J Surg Pathol.* 1996;20(7):802–814.

Robinson BD, Epstein JI. Intraductal carcinoma of the prostate without invasive carcinoma on needle biopsy: emphasis on radical prostatectomy findings. *J Urol.* 2010;184(4):1328–1333.

Shah RB, Magi-Galluzzi C, Han B, Zhou M. Atypical cribriform lesions of the prostate: relationship to prostatic carcinoma and implication for diagnosis in prostate biopsies. *Am J Surg Pathol.* 2010;34(4):470–477.

PROSTATIC DUCTAL ADENOCARCINOMA

Humphrey PA. Histological variants of prostatic carcinoma and their significance. *Histopathology.* 2012;60:59–74.

Herawi M, Epstein JI. Immunohistochemical antibody cocktail staining (p63/HMWCK/AMACR) of ductal adenocarcinoma and Gleason pattern 4 cribriform and noncribriform acinar adenocarcinomas of the prostate. *Am J Surg Pathol.* 2007;31(6):889–894.

Morgan TM, Welty CJ, Vakar-Lopez F, Lin DW, Wright JL. Ductal adenocarcinoma of the prostate: increased mortality risk and decreased serum prostate specific antigen. *J Urol.* 2010;184(6):2303–2307.

Orihuela E, Green JM. Ductal prostate cancer: contemporary management and outcomes. *Urol Oncol.* 2008;26:368.

Tavora F, Epstein JI. High-grade prostatic intraepithelial neoplasia-like ductal adenocarcinoma of the prostate: a clinicopathologic study of 28 cases. *Am J Surg Pathol.* 2008;32(7):1060–1067.

Tu SM, Lopez A, Leibovici D, et al. Ductal adenocarcinoma of the prostate: clinical features and implications after local therapy. *Cancer.* 2009;115:2872.

Samaratunga H, Letizia B. Prostatic ductal adenocarcinoma presenting as a urethral polyp: a clinicopathological study of eight cases of a lesion with the potential to be misdiagnosed as a benign prostatic urethral polyp. *Pathology.* 2007;39:476.

SMALL CELL CARCINOMA

Lotan TL, Gupta NS, Wang W, et al. ERG gene rearrangements are common in prostatic small cell carcinomas. *Mod Pathol.* 2011;24(6):820–828.

Nicholson SA, Beasley MB, Brambilla E, et al. Small cell lung carcinoma (SCLC): a clinicopathologic study of 100 cases with surgical specimens. *Am J Surg Pathol.* 2002;26(9):1184–1197.

Simon RA, di Sant'Agnese PA, Huang LS, et al. CD44 expression is a feature of prostatic small cell carcinoma and distinguishes it from its mimickers. *Hum Pathol.* 2009;40(2):252–258.

Travis W, Brambilla E, Muller-Hermelink H, Harris C. Tumors of the lung. In: Travis W. ed. *WHO Histological Classification of Tumours. Pathology and Classification of Tumors of the Lung, Pleura, Thymus and Heart.* 4th ed. Lyon, France: IARC Press; 2004.

Wang W, Epstein JI. Small cell carcinoma of the prostate. A morphologic and immunohistochemical study of 95 cases. *Am J Surg Pathol.* 2008;32(1):65–71.

Yao JL, Madeb R, Bourne P, et al. Small cell carcinoma of the prostate: an immunohistochemical study. *Am J Surg Pathol.* 2006;30(6):705–712.

PROSTATE CARCINOMA WITH SQUAMOUS CELL DIFFERENTIATION

Mohan H, Bal A, Punia RP, Bawa AS. Squamous cell carcinoma of the prostate. *Int J Urol.* 2003;10(2):114–116.

Nabi G, Ansari MS, Singh I, Sharma MC, Dogra PN. Primary squamous cell carcinoma of the prostate: a rare clinicopathological entity. Report of 2 cases and review of literature. *Urol Int.* 2001;66(4):216–219.

Okada E, Kamizaki H. Primary squamous cell carcinoma of the prostate. *Int J Urol.* 2000;7(9):347–350

Parwani AV, Kronz JD, Genega EM, Gaudin P, Chang S, Epstein JI. Prostate carcinoma with squamous differentiation: an analysis of 33 cases. *Am J Surg Pathol.* 2004;28(5):651–657.

Rahmanou F, Koo J, Marinbakh AY, Solliday MP, Grob BM, Chin NW. Squamous cell carcinoma at the prostatectomy site: squamous differentiation of recurrent prostate carcinoma. *Urology.* 1999;54(4):744.

Sarma DP, Weilbaecher TG, Moon TD. Squamous cell carcinoma of prostate. *Urology.* 1991;37(3):260–262.

UROTHELIAL CARCINOMA

Cheville JC, Dundore PA, Bostwick DG, et al. Transitional cell carcinoma of the prostate: clinicopathologic study of 50 cases. *Cancer.* 1998;82(4):703–707.

Esrig D, Freeman JA, Elmajian DA, et al. Transitional cell carcinoma involving the prostate with a proposed staging classification for stromal invasion. *J Urol.* 1996;156(3):1071–1076.

Lerner SP, Shen S. Pathologic assessment and clinical significance of prostatic involvement by transitional cell carcinoma and prostate cancer. *Urol Oncol.* 2008;26(5):481–485.

Njinou Ngninkeu B, Lorge F, Moulin P, Jamart J, Van Cangh PJ. Transitional cell carcinoma involving the prostate: a clinicopathological retrospective study of 76 cases. *J Urol.* 2003;169(1):149–152.

Shen SS, Lerner SP, Muezzinoglu B, Truong LD, Amiel G, Wheeler TM. Prostatic involvement by transitional cell carcinoma in patients with bladder cancer and its prognostic significance. *Hum Pathol.* 2006;37(6):726–734.

Tabibi A, Simforoosh N, Parvin M, et al. Predictive factors for prostatic involvement by transitional cell carcinoma of the bladder. *Urol J.* 2011;8(1):43–47.

Wood DP Jr, Montie JE, Pontes JE, VanderBrug Medendorp S, Levin HS. Transitional cell carcinoma of the prostate in cystoprostatectomy specimens removed for bladder cancer. *J Urol.* 1989;141(2):346–349.

CHAPTER 3. MESENCHYMAL, HEMATOPOIETIC, AND SECONDARY TUMORS

MESENCHYMAL TUMORS

Gaudin PB, Rosai J, Epstein JI. Sarcomas and related proliferative lesions of specialized prostatic stroma: a clinicopathologic study of 22 cases. *Am J Surg Pathol.* 1998;22(2):148–162.

Hansel DE, Herawi M, Montgomery E, Epstein JI. Spindle cell lesions of the adult prostate. *Mod Pathol.* 2007;20(1):148–158.

Herawi M, Epstein JI. Specialized stromal tumors of the prostate: a clinicopathologic study of 50 cases. *Am J Surg Pathol.* 2006;30(6):694–704.

Herawi M, Montgomery EA, Epstein JI. Gastrointestinal stromal tumors (GISTs) on prostate needle biopsy: A clinicopathologic study of 8 cases. *Am J Surg Pathol.* 2006;30(11):1389–1395.

Nagar M, Epstein JI. Epithelial proliferations in prostatic stromal tumors of uncertain malignant potential (STUMP). *Am J Surg Pathol.* 2011;35(6):898–903.

HEMATOPOIETIC MALIGNANCIES

Bostwick DG, Iczkowski KA, Amin MB, Discigil G, Osborne B. Malignant lymphoma involving the prostate: report of 62 cases. *Cancer.* 1998;83(4):732–738.

Bostwick DG, Mann RB. Malignant lymphomas involving the prostate: a study of 13 cases. *Cancer.* 1985;56(12):2932–2938.

Chu PG, Huang Q, Weiss LM. Incidental and concurrent malignant lymphomas discovered at the time of prostatectomy and prostate biopsy: a study of 29 cases. *Am J Surg Pathol.* 2005;29(5):693–699.

He H, Cheng L, Weiss LM, Chu PG. Clinical outcome of incidental pelvic node malignant B-cell lymphomas discovered at the time of radical prostatectomy. *Leuk Lymphoma.* 2007;48(10):1976–1980.

Weir EG, Epstein JI. Incidental small lymphocytic lymphoma/chronic lymphocytic leukemia in pelvic lymph nodes excised at radical prostatectomy. *Arch Pathol Lab Med.* 2003;127(5):567–572.

SECONDARY NONHEMATOPOIETIC TUMORS

Bates AW, Baithun SI. Secondary solid neoplasms of the prostate: a clinico-pathological series of 51 cases. *Virchows Arch.* 2002;440(4):392–396.

Bates AW, Baithun SI. The significance of secondary neoplasms of the urinary and male genital tract. *Virchows Arch.* 2002;440(6):640–647.

Morichetti D, Mazzucchelli R, Lopez-Beltran A, et al. Secondary neoplasms of the urinary system and male genital organs. *BJU Int.* 2009;104(6):770–776.

Index

stromal tumor of uncertain malignant
potential (STUMP), 164–167
versus benign prostatic hyperplasia stromal
nodule, 28, 166
STUMP. *See* stromal tumor of uncertain
malignant potential
sustentacular cells, 56

transitional cell metaplasia, 38–40
treatment effect
on nonneoplastic prostate, 48–51, 100–101,
104–105
on prostatic adenocarcinoma, 99–108
TTF-1, 148

uroplakin, 160
urothelial carcinoma, 155–161

versus prostatic adenocarcinoma, 160–161
urothelial carcinoma in situ (CIS), 155, 156

variant differentiation of prostatic carcinoma
atrophic variant, 112–115, 117
foamy gland variant, 36, 109–113
lymphoepithelioma-like variant, 122–124
mucinous (colloid) variant, 118–119
pleomorphic giant cell variant, 126–128
prostatic intraepithelial neoplasia (PIN)-like
PIN variant, 128–132
pseudohyperplastic variant, 116–118
sarcomatoid variant, 124–126
signet ring cell variant, 120–121

well differentiated prostatic
adenocarcinoma, 90